So Long,
Marcus Welby, M.D.

I0045940

So Long, Marcus Welby, M.D.

How Today's Health Care Is Suffocating Independent Physicians—And How Some Changed to Thrive

Steve Jacob

©Copyright 2014 by Steve Jacob. All rights reserved.

With certain exceptions, no part of this book can be reproduced in any written, electronic, recording, or photocopying without written permission of the publisher or author. The exceptions would be in the case of brief quotations embodied in the critical articles or reviews and pages where permission is specifically granted in writing by the publisher or author and where authorship/source is acknowledged in the quoted materials.

Although every precaution has been taken to verify the accuracy of the information herein, the author and publisher assume no responsibility for any errors or omissions. No liability is assumed for damages that may result from the use of information contained within.

Books may be purchased by contacting the publisher or author at: Dorsam Publishing. www.DorsamPublishing.com

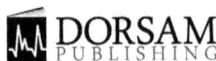

Books may be purchcased by contacting
the publisher or author at:
Dorsam Publishing
www.DorsamPublishing.com

DORSAM
PUBLISHING

Cover Design: NZ Graphics Inc.
Interior Design: Janet Long
Charts: Carol Zuber-Mallison, ZM Graphics
Editor: Peter Kaufman
Publisher: Dorsam Publishing *www.DorsamPublishing.com*

Library of Congress Catalog: #2014935949

ISBN: 978-0-9839950-2-9

1. Health Care.   2. Health Reform.   3. Health Workforce.
4. Health Costs.

First Edition. Printed in the USA.

Dedication

*To my loving and supportive family: wife Paula,
sons Ben and Joe, and daughter Megan*

Acknowledgments

This book could not have been done without the efforts of several contributors: my dogged editor Peter Kaufman; cover designer Nick Zellinger; book designer Janet Long; graphic artist Carol Zuber-Mallison and, most of all, my wife Paula. I also want to thank Lou Goodman and the board of the Physicians Foundation for their support of this project.

Table of Contents

CHAPTER 1

Introduction

A 30-ish public-relations executive representing a large, modern physician practice was shaking her head in puzzlement.

Her physician client liked to talk about how his practice was not "a Marcus Welby shop," meaning that its approach and technology reflected the best the 21st century had to offer.

As she walked a visitor toward the office-building exit, she confided, "He keeps talking about this Marcus Welby. I think it's someone he went to business school with."

Marcus Welby, the iconic primary care physician who treated patients with inexhaustible kindness and compassion, was at or near the top of the television network ratings and a staple of ABC's lineup from 1969 to 1976. *Marcus Welby, M.D.*, rose to No. 1 in the Nielsen ratings in its second season, viewed regularly in about one out of four American homes. Stars Robert Young (Welby) and James Brolin, who played partner Steven Kiley, won Emmy Awards in 1971, and Young won a Golden Globe in 1972.

Welby and Kiley became role models for many baby boomer

physicians, the leading edge of whom were graduating from medical school during the show's heyday. The pair worked hard and cared deeply about their patients—not unlike today's counterparts. Kiley was considered hipper, mostly because of his youth and the fact that he tooled around the Los Angeles suburbs on a motorcycle. Welby made house calls in a long blue sedan.

Yet Kiley seemed to take a more conventional approach to medicine, perhaps reflecting the by-the-book instincts of a recent medical school graduate. Welby, a generation or two older, was more of an out-of-the-box thinker.

The show was Hollywood's version of how medicine was practiced 40 years ago. Physicians puffed on cigarettes in the hospital boardroom, and nurses wore white uniforms and caps as they tended to patients.

Yet Welby dealt with controversial issues far removed from Young's previous Pollyanna television hit *Father Knows Best.* Story lines included rape, dementia, addiction to painkillers, depression, impotence and sexually transmitted diseases. Members of the American Academy of Family Physicians served as technical advisers for the series and reviewed scripts for accuracy.

Predictably, most diseases could be cured within the show's hour-long time slot. If not, Welby would at least ease the patient's emotional burden. Young received thousands of letters from fans asking for advice on medical or personal problems.

There was some debate at the time about whether Welby's image was good for U.S. physicians. Welby could not have been a more positive face for American medicine. However, some doctors were concerned that his tireless customer service and patient bedside manner would lead to unrealistic expectations from patients. Some even believed that Welby contributed to

IF YOU HAD YOUR CAREER TO DO OVER, WOULD YOU CHOOSE TO BE A PHYSICIAN?

Percent

NO 27%	**NO 33.5%**
YES 73%	**YES 66.5%**
2008	2012

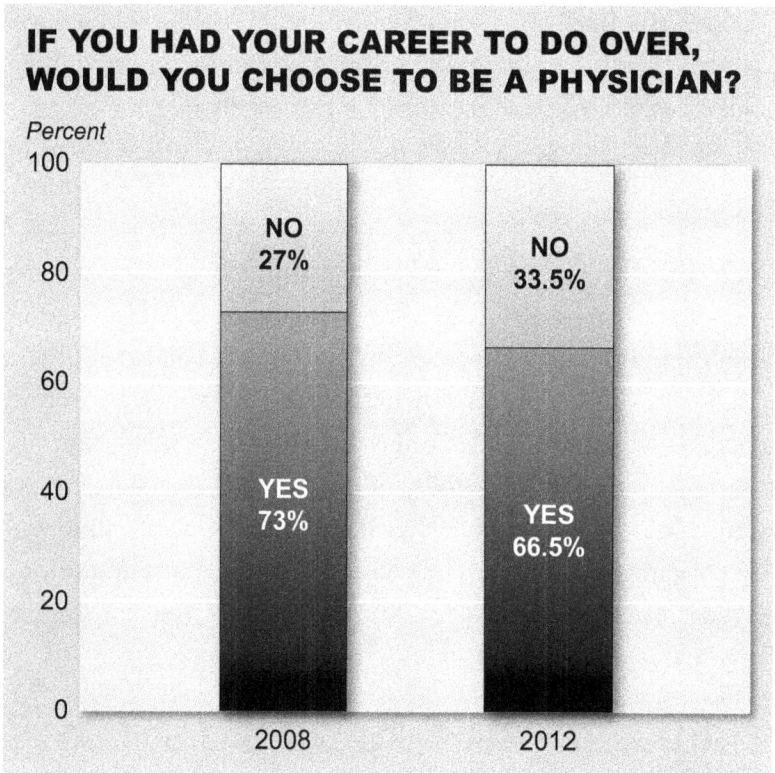

Source: Physicians Foundation Survey of America's Physicians, 2012.

More than 1 out of 3 of physicians would not choose medicine if they had their careers to do over.

the rise in malpractice lawsuits.

Young himself suffered from chemical imbalances that made him prone to depression and alcoholism. He insisted that the scripts spotlight the contribution of behavioral problems to medical conditions. Welby always seemed to address behavioral problems first, which usually greased the pathway to the cure for acute conditions.

However, the show did display its naiveté and created

controversy. In a 1973 episode, Welby advised a middle-aged man to resist his homosexual urges. The following year, an episode featured a sexual assault of a teen-age student by a male teacher that seemed to conflate homosexuality and pedophilia.

The modern-day Welby

Dr. Don McCanne, a senior health policy fellow at Physicians for a National Health Program, wrote a 2011 blog post titled, "How would Marcus Welby, M.D., fare in an ACO?"

The broader question is whether Welby would be able to function effectively under today's government regulation and insurance bureaucracy. Welby and Kiley had one nurse/receptionist. It is no wonder that they could spend so much time with the patients. The pair comprised the ultimate patient-centered medical home—no need for National Committee for Quality Assurance certification.

During the show's run in the late 1960s and early 1970s, physician payment from Medicare was based on a system of customary, prevailing and reasonable charges. From the mid-1970s through the mid-1980s, government implemented a series of cost controls. Nearly half of medical bills were paid out of pocket by commercially insured patients, compared with less than 10 percent today.

The appeal of primary care as a career seemed endless at the time. During the show's final season in 1976, a Department of Health, Education and Welfare advisory committee predicted a surplus of 145,000 primary-care physicians by 2000.

It did not work out that way. In a 2005 survey of U.S. med school seniors, half considered limits on income and lifestyle as serious obstacles to entering a primary care practice. However,

WOULD YOU RECOMMEND MEDICINE AS A CAREER TO YOUR CHILDREN OR OTHER YOUNG PEOPLE?

Percent

	2008	2012
NO	59.8%	57.9%
YES	40.2%	42.1%

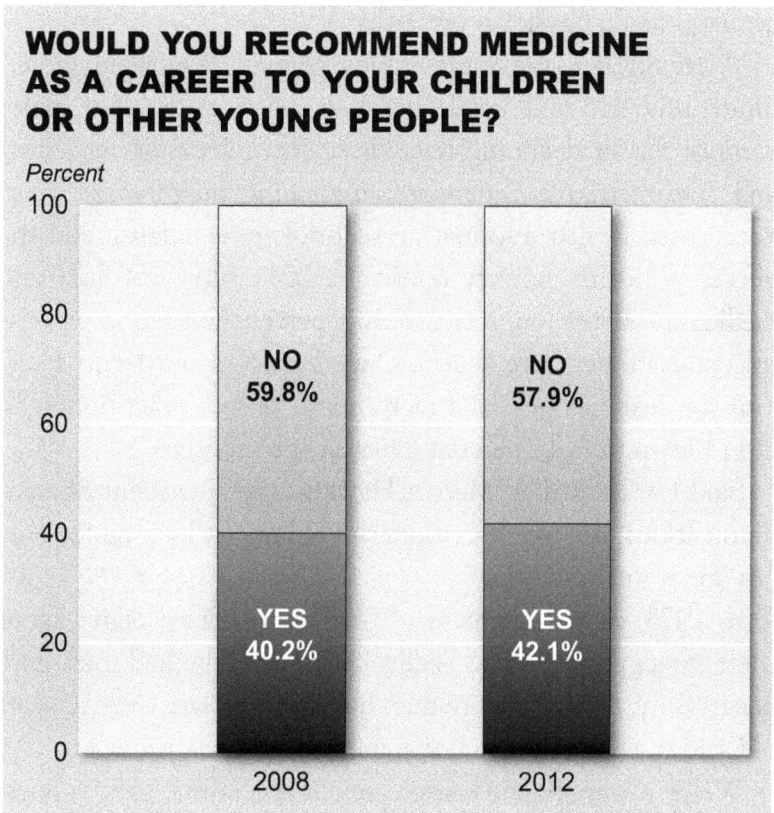

Source: Physicians Foundation Survey of America's Physicians, 2012.

A majority of physicians—nearly 58 percent—would not recommend medicine as a career to their children or other young people.

the No. 1 deterrent, respondents said, was the lack of positive role models or mentors. There were no more Marcus Welbys. Instead, about three out of four physicians between age 50 and 65 said medicine was increasingly unsatisfying, according to a 2004 survey.

Physician recruiter Merritt Hawkins CEO Mark Smith testified before a U.S. House subcommittee in July 2012 on the decline of solo physician practices.

"Virtually no one wants to be Marcus Welby anymore," Smith said. He said small physician practices face five major barriers: flat or declining reimbursement; increasing regulatory and administrative paperwork; increasing malpractice insurance costs; health information-technology mandates; and the effects of health-delivery reform. A 2011 survey of final-year medical residents found that only 1 percent wanted to work as solo practitioners like Welby. Only 2 percent of Merritt Hawkins job searches involved recruitment of solo practitioners in 2011, down from 17 percent five years previously.

Said Phillip Miller, Merritt Hawkins vice president of communications, of solo practitioners: "No one is looking for one. No one wants to be one."

In 1973, only 15 percent of physicians voiced regret about their career choice—and Welby certainly embodied that sense of certainty. By 2002, more than half of physicians over 50 years old said they would not choose medicine as a career again.

Welby always seemed suspicious of specialists, so it is questionable how skilled he would have been at care coordination. However, even he moved his practice to a hospital toward the end of the show's run.

Younger doctors want greater work-life balance

Baby boomer physicians often deride the fact that newly minted doctors want lives that are more balanced. Many older physicians still work Welby-style 70-to-80-hour weeks. White men dominated the profession in the 1970s. Fewer than 8 percent of physicians were women. Women now make up about half of incoming medical school classes. Research shows that they work fewer hours, largely because of family obligations.

Ripley Hollister, Colorado family physician and Physicians Foundation board member, said: "The older ones are being pushed out (of the system). Many are pissed off and leaving. They have a different view of medicine than the new ones. Being a doctor defined who they were. It was their purpose in life. Younger doctors work maybe 40 hours a week. They see it more as employment than a profession. They have a different view about quality of life. They won't be quite the workforce (in quantity of hours)."

Darrell Kirch, president of the Association of American Medical Colleges, believes that new physicians have a more expansive view of medicine and life, and considers that a positive development.

"I see no evidence that indicates that their ethical commitment is any weaker, that they care any less for patients," he told the Associated Press.

New Hampshire physician and Dartmouth Medical School professor Robert Wortmann wrote: "It's a bit unfair to consider Generation X physicians to be unprofessional. Times change and so does our profession. Marcus Welby did not have a working wife, a computer, a preauthorization clerk in his office, or a utilization review committee in his hospital. When he started practice, there were only two non-steroidal anti-inflammatory drugs available, and hypertension was not treated until it became symptomatic. Few hospitals had coronary-care units. Compared with today's environment, he had so few tools to work with that his most valuable patient care resource was his time."

In some ways, Welby was the predecessor of a concierge physician. He was available 24/7 and would spend as much time as the patient needed. Welby, of course, did not get a monthly re-tainer fee. In fact, he was quick to provide uncompensated care.

The spirit of Marcus Welby lives in today's physicians. However, his business model is swiftly disappearing from the American landscape. Welby's practice style could not survive financially in today's medical culture: having to see one patient every 15 minutes to keep the practice open; seeking insurance preauthorization for treatment; and being office-bound.

Declaring a full-scale revamping of health-care quality and population health while lowering costs is a daunting task. That tension is highlighted by what Yale University professor William Kissick calls "the iron triangle" of health care: quality, cost and access. Each component competes for resources at the expense of the others. Costs can be cut but, if that is done un-wisely, quality and access suffer. Access can be broadened, but it inevitably will cost more and may harm quality. Improving quality also likely will cost more and may restrict access.

Put differently, it is a version of the project management tri-angle: cheap, good, fast...pick two.

Clock is ticking on runaway health costs

There is a growing sense that, regardless of the implementa-tion of the ACA, the U.S. is running out of time to deal with the pernicious nature of health-care costs. They are approach-ing 20 percent of the U.S. economy—crowding out other government priorities, diminishing workers' wages, businesses' profits and household savings.

The current trajectory will shift more costs onto patients and employees. That is not altogether bad. Nearly two-thirds of pa-tients do not know the cost of their care until the bill shows up in the mail. The rapid increase in high-deductible plans is making patients more motivated—if not always savvier—health-care consumers. Unfortunately, most lack the tools to make intelligent choices.

Another inevitable shift is embedded in the swiftly rising increases in the cost of employer-sponsored insurance. Government will continue to squeeze Medicare and Medicaid reimbursement, leaving health-care organizations nowhere to go for additional revenue other than to American businesses.

In November 2012, a consortium of major employers and labor unions issued a manifesto of sorts demanding price transparency from health-care providers and health insurers. Consumers, they said, "have the right to know the price and quality of their health-care choices."

Billionaire investor Warren Buffett, in an interview with Bloomberg Television, called health care a tapeworm in the economy's digestive tract. "The health-care problem is the No. 1 problem of America and American business," he said. "It's the tapeworm, essentially, of the American economy, and we have not dealt with that yet."

Buffett pointed out the disadvantage U.S. businesses face in competing with companies based in nations with publicly funded, universal health plans.

Health care accounts for about 18 percent of the U.S. economy, compared with about 10 percent in other industrialized nations. Buffett said, "There's only 100 points in the dollar, and to have a 7- or 8-point disadvantage is huge. In terms of cost, it's going to require a huge change."

Many other nations are recognizing that universal health coverage for their citizens is a competitive advantage and a requirement to sustain economic growth. China is completing a three-year, $124 billion program intended to cover 90 percent of its citizens. Mexico is wrapping up an eight-year effort to provide universal coverage. Thailand, with an economy one-fifth the size of the U.S. economy, covers all but 1 percent of its population.

The endgame for many U.S. patients is to forgo some care or throw in the towel on medical bills, by either bankruptcy or ruined credit. This, too, is a distinctly American phenomenon. When other nations look at the U.S. health-care system, they cannot fathom how medical care can be the leading cause of bankruptcy in the world's richest nation.

However, all nations are facing the same thing: aging populations, mounting incidence of chronic disease and difficulty in fitting expensive medical technology within their financial means.

The U.S. health-care system combines high costs and mediocre performance, clearly pointing to great inefficiencies. Patients bear some responsibility for health outcomes by eating and smoking too much, moving too little and failing to control their blood pressure and cholesterol levels.

However, the Institute of Medicine (IOM) estimated the annual excess cost of health care to be $765 billion: $210 billion in unnecessary services, $130 billion in inefficient services, $190 billion in unneeded administrative costs, $105 billion in needlessly high prices, $55 billion in failed disease prevention and $75 billion in fraud. That $765 billion represents about 30 percent of the nation's health-care bill.

No shortage of proposed solutions

There is no shortage of proposed solutions to this mess.

WHAT TWO FACTORS DO YOU FIND LEAST SATISFYING ABOUT MEDICAL PRACTICE?

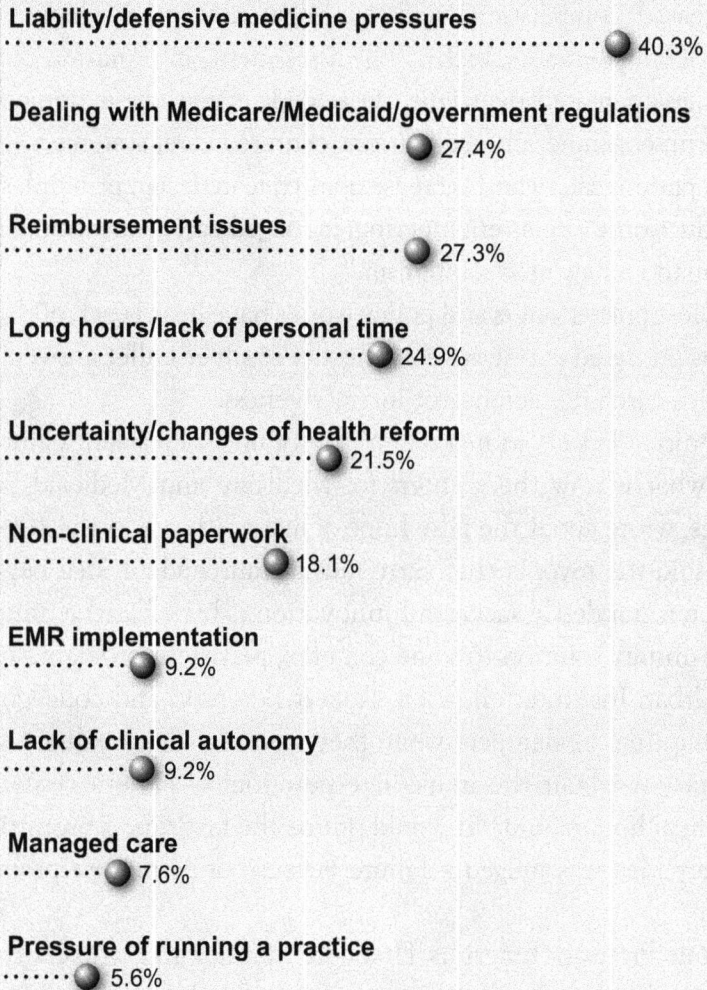

Liability/defensive medicine pressures
.... 40.3%

Dealing with Medicare/Medicaid/government regulations
.... 27.4%

Reimbursement issues
.... 27.3%

Long hours/lack of personal time
.... 24.9%

Uncertainty/changes of health reform
.... 21.5%

Non-clinical paperwork
.... 18.1%

EMR implementation
.... 9.2%

Lack of clinical autonomy
.... 9.2%

Managed care
.... 7.6%

Pressure of running a practice
.... 5.6%

Source: Physicians Foundation Survey of America's Physicians, 2012.

Physicians cite the threat of legal liability as the least satisfying aspect of practicing medicine.

Physician Harvey Fineberg, IOM president, compiled an outstanding laundry list in a 2011 lecture at the Massachusetts Medical Society: "single-payer system, an all-payer system, increased competition, reduced fragmentation, a change in physician payments, technology assessment, information technology, increased oversight, decreased regulation, malpractice reform, consumer choice, patient-centered care, systems to ensure patient safety and increase quality, lean design principles of production, systems engineering, managed care, educational reform and a new professionalism."

Most practitioners and policy wonks have heard each of these ideas proffered at one time or another as silver-bullet answers to health care's inefficiency or ineffectiveness.

Bruce Vladeck, former administrator under President Clinton for what is now the Centers for Medicare and Medicaid Services, wrote about the false hope of managed care in the 1990s. He said the myopia that surrounds a transcendent idea begins when a "modestly successful innovation is hyped as the unique and unitary solution to some complex, persistent problem."

Urban Institute fellow Dr. Robert Berenson and colleagues, attempting to dampen what they considered unrealistic expectations about the immediate potential of patient-centered medical homes, said, "It would not be the first time a promising policy idea was judged a failure because of premature promotion."

Yale Professor Emeritus Theodore Marmor and University of North Carolina Professor Jonathan Oberlander are even blunter about these seemingly simple solutions: "The United States has been singularly unsuccessful at controlling health-care spending. During the past four decades, American policymakers and analysts have embraced an ever-changing array of panaceas to control costs, including managed care, consumer-directed health care, and most recently, delivery system reform and value-based purchasing.

"Past panaceas have gone through a cycle of excessive hope followed by disappointment at their failure to rein in medical-care spending…[A]ccountable care organizations, medical homes, and similar ideas in vogue today could repeat this pattern…[T]he United States persistently pursues health policy fads—despite their poor record—and the promotion of panaceas obscures critical debate about controlling health-care costs. Americans spend too much time on the quest for the 'holy grail'—a reform that will decisively curtail spending while simultaneously improving quality of care—and too little time learning from the experiences of others. Reliable cost control does not, contrary to conventional wisdom, require fundamental delivery system reform or an end to fee-for-service payment. It does require the U.S. to emulate the lessons of other nations that have been more successful at limiting spending through budgeting, system-wide fee schedules, and concentrated purchasing."

They conclude that "the American quest for cost-control fads hasn't worked—which helps explain why the U.S. keeps searching for more panaceas."

While medical costs are becoming stratospheric, physicians generally are not to blame. As a rule of thumb, a 30-20-10 percent ratio reflects the proportion of health-care costs that go to hospitals, physicians and prescription drugs. However, it is medical technology and the market power of large health-care organizations that are driving the increases. From 1974 to 2010, the number of U.S. patents granted for pharmaceutical and surgical innovations increased sixfold.

The percentage of medical bills paid directly by the patient has declined significantly over the past 50 years because almost no one can afford adequate health care without being subsidized by the government or an employer. Despite this, rising health-care costs have eliminated any appreciable gains in income for American families. The average household income rose from $76,000 to $99,000 from 1999 to 2009. Health-care cost increases wiped out all but $95 per month of that increase. If medical inflation had matched the general rate of inflation as measured by the Consumer Price Index, the average family would have had $545 more a month to spend or save.

More influence than income

Meanwhile, physicians have to fight for every dollar. Plumbers and attorneys do not have to call a third party to verify that they will be paid when they fix leaky faucets or draw up wills. Primary-care physicians' share of the U.S. health-care dollar is only 7 cents. If payers cut reimbursement for physician services by 25 percent, the average annual rate of medical inflation would only decrease to 5.7 percent from 6.2 percent. However, primary-care doctors control 80 cents of the health-care dollar by sending their patients to hospitals, referring them to specialists and handing out prescriptions.

This outsize influence extends to patient perceptions. Nurses, pharmacists and physicians annually occupy the top three spots in the annual Gallup survey of how Americans gauge honesty and ethics among professions. Gallup has polled on public trust in professionals since 1976. In its 2012 survey, nurses scored the highest, at 85 percent on "honesty and ethical standards," followed by pharmacists at 80 percent and physicians at 70 percent.

More than three out of four Americans say their physicians put patients' interests ahead of their own, according to a Kaiser Family Foundation poll.

About four out of 10 Americans say they are confident in the U.S. health-care system, but more than eight out of 10 say the health care they receive personally is good or excellent. Physicians are seen as heroes who help people when they are sick, not as cogs in an impersonal economic sector.

Cardiologist Rick Snyder, former president of the Dallas County Medical Society, says physicians do not advocate on their own behalf and fail to use their considerable influence.

"By being an advocate you can treat a whole state or country, not just one patient," Snyder said. "What are the most credible professions? Nurses and doctors. (Republican pollster) Frank Luntz once said, 'You doctors are God and the law.' "

Stanford University professors Victor Fuchs and Arnold Milstein agree. They wrote in the New England Journal of Medicine, "...Physicians are the most influential element in health care. The public's trust in them makes physicians the only plausible catalyst of policies to accelerate diffusion of cost-effective care. Are U.S. physicians sufficiently visionary, public-minded and well led to respond to this national fiscal and ethical imperative?"

Unfortunately, the annual battle to avoid reimbursement cuts because of Medicare's sustainable growth rate has absorbed physicians' attention in the political arena. All other issues pale by comparison.

Only 15 percent of U.S. primary-care physicians believe the nation's health-care system works well. More than half are frustrated by the difficulty many of their patients face in paying for care.

Burnout is pervasive

According to a large study in 2012, nearly half of U.S. physicians struggle with job burnout. They said they either were emotionally exhausted or felt a high degree of cynicism or "depersonalization" toward their patients.

The researchers used a questionnaire called the Maslach Burnout Inventory, considered the best measure of job burnout. Burnout was especially prevalent among physicians on the front lines of medicine, such as those who staff emergency rooms or family practices.

On average, physicians worked about 10 hours a week more than other professionals—50 hours vs. the standard 40—and more than one out of three worked more than 60 hours a week. More than four out of 10 expressed dissatisfaction with their work-life balance, almost double the rate of non-physicians.

The study's authors struck this disheartening note: "Unfortunately, little evidence exists about how to address this problem. Policymakers and health-care organizations must address the problem of burnout for the sake of physicians and their patients."

A separate survey found that 86 percent of physicians are moderately to severely stressed. Respondents said their top four stress factors were the economy, health-care reform, Medicare and Medicaid policies, and patients without the means to pay for their care.

Physicians have the highest suicide rate of any profession, for distinctive reasons. Non-physicians are more likely to have had a specific traumatic event, such as a personal crisis or death of a loved one. Physicians are more likely to have on-the-job stress or a specific professional problem. They also are less likely to undergo mental-health treatment.

A study of surgeons with work-home conflicts found they were more likely to fall prey to alcohol abuse and depression because of poor work-life balance. The average surgeon works 60 hours a week, spends 16 of those hours in the operating room and is on call two nights a week. About half who reported work-life conflicts showed signs of depression while more than one out of six of those showed signs of alcohol abuse or dependency.

Physician burnout starts early. Nearly half of medical students become burned out during their training. Students are overworked, fearful of making mistakes and encouraged to tamp down emotions such as grief and self-doubt.

It is troubling that the nation's health is in the hands of a profession that displays such pervasive signs of disaffection, disenfranchisement and hopelessness.

Even young physicians exhibit a high degree of pessimism. An April 2012 Physicians Foundation survey of physicians under 40 found that more than half were pessimistic about the future of the U.S. health-care system, while 22 percent were optimistic.

Those physicians who are satisfied with their profession tend to display an evangelist's zeal for practicing medicine, and enjoy addressing conditions such as obesity and nicotine or alcohol dependence. Their empathy also translates into better patient outcomes. *Academic Medicine* researchers used a Jefferson Scale of Empathy (JSE), designed in 2001 to measure empathy in a medical setting. They found a direct association between a positive physician JSE score and better control of patients' hemoglobin A1c and cholesterol levels. Pure and simple, physician satisfaction translates into better patient health.

A survey of hospital executives and practice managers by physician recruiting firm Merritt Hawkins underscores the sharp contrast in the outlook of health-care executives compared with that of physicians. Merritt Hawkins surveyed U.S. physicians for the Physicians Foundation in 2012.

- More than nine out of 10 executives say they feel positive about being in health-care management, compared with one out of three physicians who say they feel positive about being in medicine.

- Nearly nine out of 10 executives say their morale is positive and they would recommend health-care management as a career, compared with about four out of 10 physicians who would make such a recommendation.

Travis Singleton, a Merritt Hawkins' senior vice president, said in a statement, "For health-care facility managers, the glass appears to be half full. For physicians, it appears to be half empty."

According to a survey by locum tenens staffing firm Staff Care, virtually all nurse practitioners said they had positive feelings about being an N.P., and 98 percent said they were optimistic about the future of their profession. In the Physicians Foundation survey, only 13 percent of physicians felt optimistic about the future of medicine.

Marcus Welby took joy in his work. But he also did not face the obstacles and pressures today's physicians must endure.

About this book

This book is based on the Physicians Foundation's top watch issues for 2013. However, these issues are long-standing and will extend well into the future.

Chapter 2 provides a broader view of the economy and explores how it affects physician practices. A slowly mending economy is lifting spending on physician services, which is expected to accelerate as the ACA's afterburners ignite in 2014. However, the increase will be a far cry from those of 2001 to 2003, which were well north of 8 percent annually. In 2011, health-care costs grew more slowly than costs in other economic sectors for the first time in more than a decade. There are no clear answers on why, or on whether the slowdown is temporary or permanent.

Chapter 3 examines how rising medical expenses are consuming a growing proportion of household budgets. The ACA is unlikely to alter that. The rise of high-deductible health plans is leading patients to forgo health care in equal amounts of necessary and unnecessary care. The plans are also putting more pressure on physician-practice revenue cycles.

Chapter 4 details the high stakes of getting patients engaged in their health. Physicians can improve patients' health only if the patients are willing to do their part. An engaged patient consistently does what needs to be done to gain the greatest benefit from available health resources. Too many patients are not holding up their end of the bargain.

Chapter 5 explores the uneasiness in the physician community over the effects of the ACA. Physicians are shying away from talking to their patients about the law. Nonetheless, patients consider physicians and nurses the most trusted sources of information. Ezekiel Emanuel, chair of medical ethics and health policy at the University of Pennsylvania, calls physicians the most important group in determining the future of the U.S. health-delivery reform. Despite the fact that most physicians did not favor the ACA, its success or failure rests on their weary shoulders.

Chapter 6 chronicles the dizzying pace at which hospitals are gobbling physician practices to secure referrals, create accountable care organizations and seize greater control over quality initiatives. Physicians are seeking out the security and stable income of employment while struggling to maintain as much autonomy as possible. Hospitals are merging with one another as well, as everyone tries to become big to compete under delivery reform. Newly merged hospitals are raising prices by as much as 40 percent.

Chapter 7 considers the folly of insuring nearly 30 million more Americans in 2014 without expanding the provider base. The U.S. already has a shortage of more than 15,000 primary-care physicians, and hospital emergency visits are rising at twice the rate of population growth. Another 7,000 primary-care physicians would be needed to treat those who are expected to gain insurance for the first time in 2014.

Chapter 8 recounts the factors that are sapping physician autonomy. In a survey, physicians cite decreasing independence as their greatest source of dissatisfaction, ahead of declining reimbursement and administrative hassles. Rising practice expenses, unrealistic demands from patients, government mandates, medical liability and time pressures conspire to keep physicians from doing what they want to do most: deliver high-quality patient care.

Chapter 9 explains the plethora of time-eating administrative burdens physicians face. More than three out of four physicians believe insurers use excessive preauthorization for tests, procedures and medications. Physicians spend about 20 percent of their workday in activities outside the exam room. The average physician spends a total of nearly three weeks per year dealing with health plans. In addition, 23 weeks of nursing staff time and 44 weeks of clerical staff time are spent on insurance claims.

Chapter 10 explores some possible ways for physicians to remain independent, and profiles some physicians who are thriving by using new practice models.

CHAPTER 2

The "Physician" Economy

S pending on physician services grew by 3.6 percent in 2011, compared with 2.8 percent the previous year. However, rate of growth is well short of when increases were more than 8 percent annually a decade earlier.

During the economic downturn in 2009 and 2010, health-care costs grew at their slowest rate in decades. According to the Centers for Medicare and Medicaid Services (CMS) Office of the Actuary, health-care spending grew by 3.9 percent for the third consecutive year in 2011.

Health-care costs grew more slowly than the rest of the economy in 2011, for the first time in more than a decade. For health policy analysts, that is huge: When they call for aggressive cost controls, they usually urge cost growth that is one percentage point higher than the rest of the economy. That, for example, is the target for Medicare cost growth in the Affordable Care Act (ACA). If Medicare costs grow any faster than that, the Independent Payment Advisory Board is directed to make binding recommendations to Congress on the best way to hit that target.

Probably the biggest economic question hanging over health care is whether the recent slowdown in spending growth is permanent or temporary.

Three major studies have agreed that the recent recession contributed to the slowdown, but to varying degrees.

A Kaiser Family Foundation study estimated that the recession accounted for about 75 percent of the spending restraint, while the other 25 percent was due to noneconomic factors.

David Cutler, a Harvard health economist, estimated that the recession accounted for slightly more than one-third of the slowdown.

And the third study, by Harvard Medical School professor Michael Chernew, pointed to rising out-of-pocket consumer costs as responsible for about 20 percent of the decline in health spending. Other factors, he found, included less rapid development of new prescription drugs and the movement from fee-for-service to value-based reimbursement.

The Chernew study underscores the fact that households are feeling the increasing burden of health-care costs despite the slowdown in medical inflation.

"The slowdown in health costs is completely unreal to average people," Drew Altman, the president of the Kaiser Family Foundation, told *The New York Times.* "Experts measure aggregate spending. But people's (medical) costs have gone up 140 percent over the past 10 years, while wages only went up 40 percent."

Health-care spending growth was expected to remain under 4 percent in 2013 because of the sluggish economic recovery, continued increases in cost-sharing requirements for the privately insured, and slow growth for Medicare and Medicaid spending.

WHAT ARE MAJOR DRIVERS CONTRIBUTING TO RISING HEALTH COSTS?

Defensive medicine
.... 69.1%

Aging population
.... 64.9%

Cost of pharmaceuticals
.... 59.1%

Advances in technology/treatment
.... 51.2%

**Social conditions
(poverty, drugs, violence, illegal immigration, etc.)**
.... 43.5%

State and federal insurance mandates
.... 41.6%

Lack of pricing transparency
.... 40.5%

Limited patient financial obligations
.... 39%

Absence of free markets
.... 37.2%

Fraud
.... 18.8%

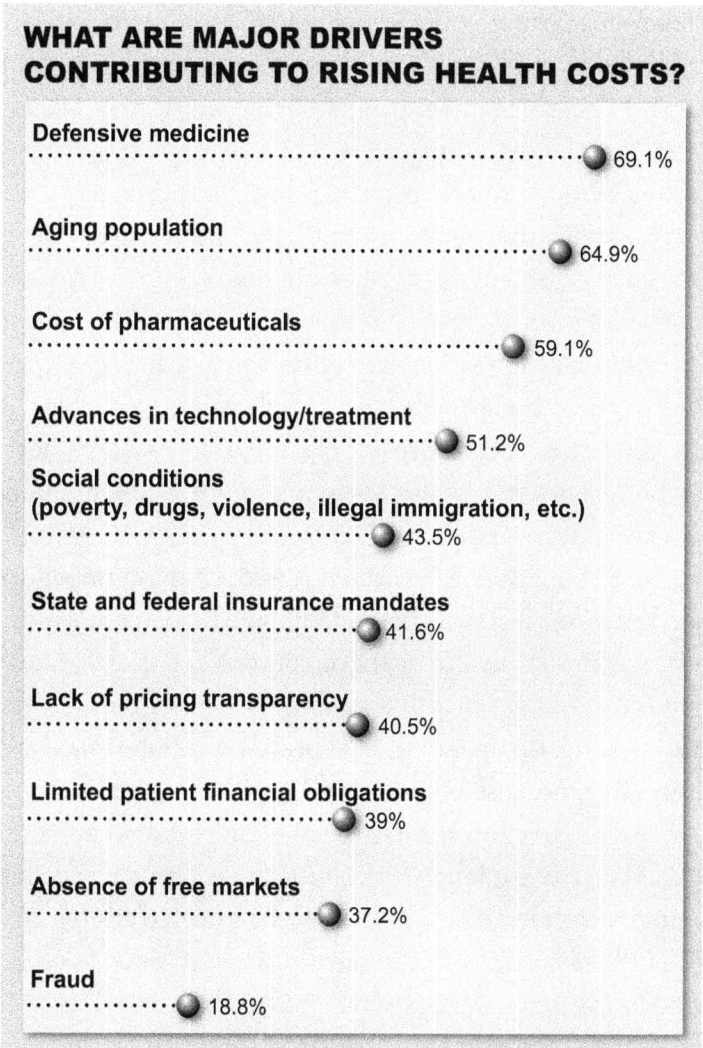

Source: Physicians Foundation Survey of America's Physicians, 2012.

Nearly 7 out of 10 physicians say defensive medicine is a key driver of health-care costs.

However, starting in 2014, overall growth in national health spending is expected to accelerate to 6.1 percent, reflecting expanded insurance coverage under the ACA, through either Medicaid or the marketplaces. The use of medical services and goods, especially prescription drugs and physician and clinical services among the newly insured, is expected to contribute significantly to spending increases of more than 12 percent in Medicaid and nearly 8 percent under private health insurance.

"Primary-care physicians are often the first point of contact within the health-care system for people gaining coverage. As a result, the newly insured are anticipated to devote a higher proportion of their total health spending to physician and clinical services," CMS actuaries said.

By 2022, the ACA is projected to reduce the number of uninsured people by 30 million, add about 0.1 percentage points to average annual health spending growth for those years, and increase cumulative health spending by $621 billion. Growth in national health spending is expected to remain near 6 percent in 2015, because of two main factors. First, 8 million more Americans will gain insurance coverage that year through Medicaid or the exchanges. Second, the economic recovery is expected to accelerate in 2014-15, with projected annual growth in the GDP exceeding 5 percent for the first time since 2006. The resulting gains in disposable personal income should drive increased use of health-care goods and services.

Medicare expenditures are projected to grow by an average of 7.9 percent per year from 2019 to 2022, compared with 7.3 percent per year between 2016 and 2018, as baby boomers continue to enroll in the program. An additional 8.8 million people are projected to enroll in Medicaid by 2016, because some additional states are expected to expand their Medicaid programs after 2014.

By 2022, federal, state, and local governments are projected to account for 49 percent of total national health expenditures, reaching a total of $2.4 trillion. The federal government is expected to account for more than 63 percent of that total.

The yin and yang of costs and utilization

Payers that focus on controlling prices often fail, because providers ramp up utilization in response.

Conversely, those attempting to keep expenditures down by managing utilization often falter because of relentless cost growth. Medicare and Medicaid set prices administratively to curb costs. However, Dartmouth researchers have shown that two-thirds of the geographical variation in Medicare spending stems from differences in service volume.

Commercial insurers have concentrated on controlling the quantity of care delivered, primarily through greater cost sharing and capitation payments. According to the Health Care Cost Institute (HCCI), one of the largest financial databases for the private marketplace, utilization decreased significantly between 2007 and 2010. However, in 2009 and 2010, per-capita health-care costs in working-age adults were driven almost entirely by price increases for services.

The ratio of private-payer rates to hospitals' service-delivery costs increased from 116 percent in 2000 to 134 percent in 2009. Meanwhile, the ratio of Medicare payment to service cost declined from about 100 percent to 90 percent.

Many major health systems traditionally exercised market power to extract higher payment rates from private insurers.

The cost shifting from government insurance programs that often do not cover the cost of care had become an accepted practice in health-care financing.

However, there is evidence that hospitals are no longer relying on cost shifting. A 2013 *Health Services Research* study of 13 years of hospital cost reports concluded that nonprofit hospitals cut operating costs to adjust to reduced revenues, while for-profit hospitals—which already have lower operating costs—likely would see profits decline.

Research shows that Medicare cuts actually result in lower rates paid by private payers. A *Health Affairs* study found that a 10 percent Medicare rate reduction was associated with a 7.73 percent reduction in payments from private insurers. A study of Florida outpatient surgical hospitals found that Medicare rate cuts resulted in a higher volume of procedures from private payers, which suggests the hospitals lowered their private rates to attract more business and offset the Medicare losses.

As recipients of medical spending, physicians are no longer king of the hill. According to the Milliman Medical Index, the physician slice of health-care spending by a family of four has shrunk from 37 percent in 2005 to 32 percent in 2012. Meanwhile, the shares of inpatient and outpatient care have grown to 32 percent and 18 percent, respectively.

The bigger problem is that reimbursement is being eclipsed by physician practice expenses, such as staff salaries, health insurance, malpractice expenses and technology acquisition. According to the Medical Group Management Association (MGMA), practice revenue grew 45 percent between 2001 and 2010, while practice expenses rose 53 percent—despite a decline of more than 2 percent in 2010 as practices aggressively

GROWTH OF SPENDING ON PHYSICIAN SERVICES

Percent

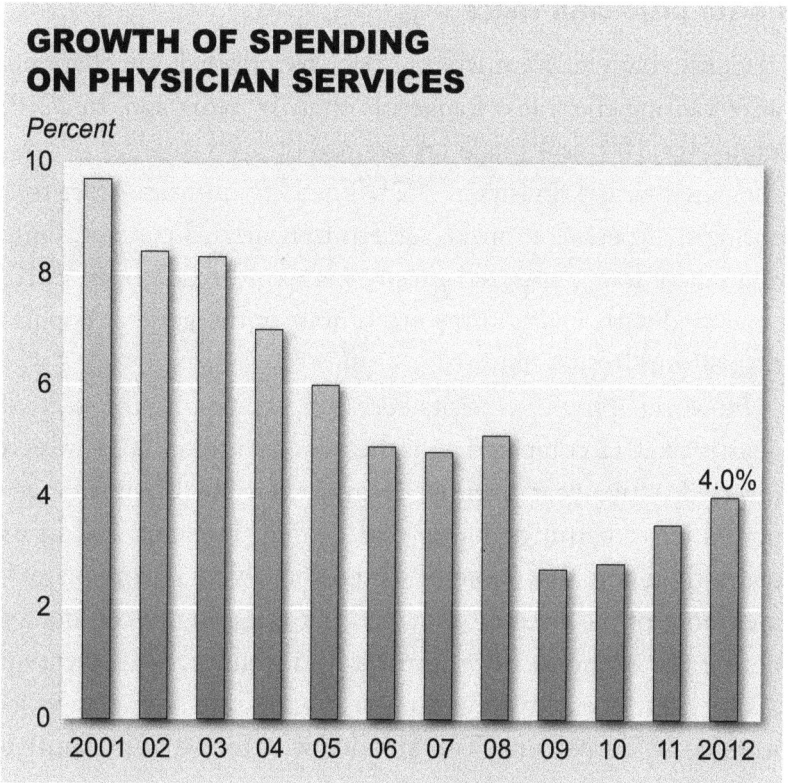

Bar chart showing growth of spending on physician services by year: 2001 ~9.7, 02 ~8.4, 03 ~8.3, 04 ~7.0, 05 ~6.0, 06 ~4.8, 07 ~4.7, 08 ~5.1, 09 ~2.6, 10 ~2.7, 11 ~3.4, 2012 4.0%

Source: Centers for Medicare and Medicaid. Office of the Actuary.

Growth of spending on physician services increased for three straight years after a nose dive during the Great Recession.

cut spending that final year.

PricewaterhouseCoopers (PwC) predicted slow growth on physician spending in 2013. PwC said physicians would face stiffer competition from proliferating alternative-care competitors, such as retail and workplace clinics, telemedicine and mobile health tools.

Fewer physician visits

Census data bear out what physicians already know: Patients were visiting them less frequently than 10 years ago. In 2010, adults age 18 to 64 made an average of 3.9 visits per person, compared with 4.8 visits in 2001. The U.S. uninsured rate rose during that period, from 17 percent to nearly 22 percent. Only one out of four uninsured people went to the doctor in 2010, compared with nearly three out of four of the general population of working adults.

However, physician visits rose 4.8 percent in the second quarter of 2012 compared with the same quarter in 2011, which reversed a two-year decline. Nearly every health insurer reported lower earnings during that quarter. Humana said in its quarterly report that more of its members were seeking care—and more of it—because they had put off going to the doctor during the economic downturn. It said wellness visits were up 200 percent over the previous year, and routine physician visits were up by 22 percent. The first-dollar coverage of preventive care also was a fueling factor.

Rising insurance premium costs for 2014 because of the ACA's ban on pre-existing condition underwriting and more comprehensive policies—combined with rapidly growing high-deductible insurance plans—may short-circuit the rebound in physician visits.

Even so, any rebound is welcome. Physician-office visits had declined 4.7 percent in 2011 and 4.2 percent in 2010, and had declined in four of the previous five years.

A Stanford University analysis for the Kaiser Family Foundation found a 17 percent decline in office visits between 2009 and 2011. Office visits had risen from 140 million to 160 million between 2000 and 2005 and held at that rate until the start of the recession in late 2007. The rate dropped below 130 million visits in the second quarter of 2011.

More than nine million people lost health insurance coverage during the recession. Fewer than half of unemployed adults had health insurance, compared with more than 81 percent of employed adults. Unemployed adults have poorer mental and physical health, yet they are less likely to receive needed medical care, because of cost.

Even people with private insurance have been cutting back on routine care. Rising deductibles and co-payments make people more reluctant to seek care, even if they have chronic conditions. Employees with high-deductible health plans are three to four times more likely to delay or forgo care, compared with those in more traditional plans.

The share of employees with an annual deductible of at least $1,000 grew from 18 percent in 2008 to 31 percent to 2011.

Fewer office visits also helped slow prescription drug spending. The number of prescriptions filled grew only 1.2 percent in 2012.

Slowing cost growth predates recession

The slowing rate of health-care cost growth dates back to 2001, indicating that there are other influences beside the recent recession and sluggish recovery.

Health-care costs are driven by service volume and prices. Most still suspect the recession is the major culprit in holding down growth. Millions lost employer-sponsored insurance between 2008 and 2010. Meanwhile, high-deductible plan enrollment soared, making people more reluctant to encounter the health-care system because of increased financial exposure

to the cost of care. In fact, nearly half of those who were employed throughout the recession avoided seeking some needed
care.

Even so, health-care spending did rise faster than the overall
economy during most of the past decade. Researchers point to
four primary reasons for this:

- The development and deployment of medical technology;
- Increased prevalence of chronic disease and the rising costs
  of its treatment;
- Growing consolidation and lack of competition among insurers and providers;
- Consumers' being shielded from the true cost of care by
  employer and public insurance.

Employers held health-benefit cost growth to 4.1 percent in
2012, which was the lowest in 15 years. They have stepped up
cost management in anticipation of added cost pressures from
health reform. Many health-reform opponents expected more
businesses to stop offering health insurance. According to business consultant Mercer, that number actually rose slightly in
2012.

Experts say there are too little data to determine whether
the slower increase in health-care spending is permanent or a
temporary function of the weak economy.

Harvard economist David Cutler told *The New York Times*,
"The recession just doesn't account for the numbers we're seeing. I think there's much more going on."

Economist Gail Wilensky, who headed the CMS under President George W. Bush, said, "If there's something else going
on, we don't know what it is yet. The most honest thing to say
is that, one, the reduction in use is greater than the recession

predicts; two, we don't understand why yet; and three, you'd be foolhardy to say that we can understand it."

According to the Center for Economic and Policy Research, the U.S. would have long-term budget surpluses rather than deficits if per-person health-care costs mirrored those of the rest of the world. Based on its online calculator, the U.S. deficit would be erased by 2040 if it had the same health-care prices as Australia.

During the recession, the percentage of Americans with private insurance decreased to less than 65 percent—the lowest level in 20 years.

There has been a deceleration of health-spending growth for the past eight years. Year-over-year growth declined from 9.5 percent in 2002 to 3.9 percent in 2010. The result of this trend is that Americans spent nearly $200 billion less on health care between 2006 and 2009 than they would have if the spending growth had equaled the three years prior to that.

Costs grew five times faster than the economy

U.S. health spending has grown faster than the gross domestic product annually since 1960, with the exception of eight years. The cumulative effect is that national health expenditures over those decades have grown nearly five times as much as the economy, adjusted for inflation.

Although health spending usually grows faster than the economy, its share of the U.S. economy remained at 17.9 percent in 2009 and 2010 .

The federal government took on a larger share of health-care spending as the economy slackened. As consumers, employers, and state and local governments trimmed health-care expenses, the federal government increased its health spending by 40 percent from 2007 to 2010. Much of that increase was in Medicaid, in which enrollment swelled as unemployment grew and the 2009 economic stimulus law buttressed sagging state budgets.

Health costs reached another historic benchmark in July 2010: They actually fell 0.1 percent, the first monthly decline in 35 years.

Still, health spending is rising faster than the rates of incomes and other consumer prices in most developed nations, raising worldwide concern about how future medical costs will be met.

Health-care spending has slowed worldwide. From 2000 to 2009, health spending grew by an average of 5 percent annually in 34 countries in the Organization for Economic Cooperation and Development (OECD). In 2010, there was zero growth, and OECD expects a similar result in 2011. Much of this was driven by brute-force cuts among European nations imposing austerity budgets.

Annual per-person spending, adjusted for inflation, has exceeded U.S. income growth by an average of about 2 percentage points for the past 50 years. The U.S. spends more per capita than any other nation, and its costs are rising the fastest.

The U.S. spent 17.9 percent of its GDP, or $8,650 per person, on health care in 2011. In contrast, food and housing costs each represent 10 percent of GDP. In European nations, the figure was about $3,000 per person and an average of 9 percent of GDP on health care. CMS predicts spending of $13,710 per American by 2020—nearly 20 percent of GDP.

Peter Orszag, then-director of the Congressional Budget Office (CBO), said in congressional testimony in 2007, "The nation's long-term fiscal balance will be determined primarily by the future of health-care cost growth."

Federal health-care spending is expected to more than double in the next 10 years, according to the CBO. Entitlement programs, which include Medicare and Medicaid, are projected to grow from $847 billion to $1.8 trillion in fiscal year 2022. That figure represents about 7 percent of the entire economy. The CBO cites the aging population as the major driver of federal health-care spending. Medicare is expected to grow by 90 percent—and that includes the sustainable growth-rate cuts that Congress has prevented in recent years.

Like the CBO, S&P cites the aging populations in the U.S. and elsewhere as a major reason for the danger to public finances during the first half of the 21st century. Absent reforms (and the ACA is unlikely to be a factor in curbing costs), S&P plans credit downgrades sometime in the next three years. S&P said technology accounts for up to two-thirds of projected health-care increases in its forecast.

The current trend is sobering. Health-care spending is on track to consume 119 to 142 percent of current per-capita federal spending over the next 75 years. That means health care would crowd out other valuable areas of the budget, such as national defense, Social Security and education.

This would happen despite the fact that the U.S. population is smoking less, suffering fewer heart attacks and living longer, healthier lives.

More taxes, or fewer benefits?

Former Federal Reserve Chairman Ben Bernanke warned that Americans would have to either allow higher taxes or change Medicare and Social Security in order to keep budget deficits from suffocating economic growth. The two programs account for about one-third of U.S. government spending.

Americans clearly do not like budget deficits, but they do not want to alter these revered entitlements, either. More than three-quarters of U.S. adults say it is unacceptable to cut either Social Security or Medicare. About half believe neither program needs to be cut to balance the budget. Even 70 percent of Tea Party members oppose cutting Medicare.

Part of this wishful thinking reflects how misinformed Americans are about the nation's budget. Two-thirds erroneously believe the federal government spends more on defense and foreign aid than it does on Medicare and Social Security. A majority believes the budget can be balanced by eliminating "waste, fraud and abuse." They believe an average of 43 cents of every dollar is wasted. In one poll, people were asked to estimate what percentage of the federal budget is spent on foreign aid. The average response was 27 percent. The actual amount is less than 1 percent. In 2008, just 0.19 percent of the overall GDP was spent on foreign aid, which was last among a list of 22 wealthy nations. The average wealthy nation contributed more than twice that rate. (Foreign aid excludes military deployments and "nation-building" efforts by the U.S. military.)

Employment in the health-care sector continues to be robust, despite a lagging economy. From late 2007 to February 2011, heath-care employment grew 6.3 percent. In all other sectors, employment contracted 6.8 percent. One out of nine U.S. workers is now employed in health care.

Health care and social-assistance jobs are expected to account for one out of four new jobs created by 2020. Moreover, that may be an underestimation, because of the impact of health reform. During the first five years of its health-reform initiative,

Massachusetts health-care employment grew by 9.5 percent, compared with 5.5 percent in other states. That higher rate represented 18,000 more health-care jobs.

The nature of those jobs suggests reform's increasing administrative burden. From 2005 to 2010, Massachusetts health-care administration jobs grew by 18 percent, compared with 8 percent elsewhere. Meanwhile, physician and nurse employment in the state grew by 6 and 3 percent, respectively.

Yet there are economic storm clouds on the horizon, likely the result of the ACA's reduction of Medicare reimbursement and uncompensated-care subsidies to hospitals. More than 41,000 health-care jobs were slashed in the first nine months of 2013, and the field had more layoffs than in any other economic sector in September of that year. Likewise, the health-care sector led all other industries in CEO turnover during the same period—signaling C-suite difficulty in adjusting to delivery reform.

The dreaded Sustainable Growth Rate

Commercial health plans are difficult to deal with, but at least they represent revenue that is not subject to annual legislated reduction.

The average physician practice relies on Medicare for about 25 percent of its revenue. That revenue source is at risk every year because of the Sustainable Growth Rate (SGR), established in 1997 to keep Medicare from growing faster than the overall economy. The SGR formula factored in the rising number of people on Medicare. However, the per-beneficiary costs charged by providers rose at a faster rate than the economy. When that happens, the federal government is supposed to cut payments across the board to control costs. Every year since 2002, Congress has blocked these cuts. The proposed cumulative rate cut to satisfy the SGR was scheduled to be 24 percent had Congress not stepped in again in March 2014.

According to CMS actuaries, that cut would drop Medicare pay rates to 61 percent of what private insurers pay for the same services, and even drop below those of Medicaid. Rates are scheduled to drop further until, in 2050, Medicare falls below 40 percent of what private insurers pay. The actuaries acknowledge it is unlikely that Congress would allow this scenario to play out. The annual threat of a proposed rate cut will continue until Congress fixes the formula.

Congress has overridden the SGR-mandated cuts a dozen times, substituting either pay freezes or small pay increases. The price tag for freezing physician rates has dropped significantly because of declines in health-care spending growth. According to a 2013 CBO report, the estimated 10-year cost of repealing the SGR and freezing Medicare payments to physicians would be $116.5 billion, compared with the previous estimate of $244 billion.

Nevertheless, four former Medicare administrators told a Senate committee hearing in May 2012 that the SGR must be replaced.

The American Medical Association (AMA) and more than 100 state and specialty medical societies issued a set of principles in October 2012 that they said could support a transition from the SGR to "a higher-performing Medicare program." They urged a plan that would allow physicians to choose their own payment models, eschewed penalties and allowed physicians to demonstrate that they are taking accountability for quality and cost control.

In October 2013, the Medicare Payment Advisory Commission (MedPAC) recommended eliminating the SGR formula by cutting fees for some specialists and imposing a 10-year freeze on rates for primary-care physicians. Predictably, the proposal was strongly opposed by health industry groups and the AMA.

Reps. Allyson Schwartz, D-Pa., and Joe Heck, R-Nev., an osteopathic physician, reintroduced legislation in February 2013 to repeal the SGR, increase payments to physicians for four years and test new payment and delivery models.

Alternatively, House Republican leaders have urged an SGR repeal plan that would freeze physician payment rates for the next decade, with future increases based on physicians' quality and efficiency of care.

Health-care industry groups urged Congress to use projected Iraqi and Afghanistan war savings to repeal the SGR.

In its 2013 annual report, MedPAC said, "The SGR formula may have resulted in lower reimbursement updates, but it has failed to restrain volume growth; in fact, for some specialties the formula may have exacerbated growth. In addition, the temporary increases, or 'fixes,' to override the SGR formula are undermining the credibility of Medicare by engendering uncertainty and frustration among providers, which may be causing anxiety among beneficiaries."

Nearly all lawmakers want to repeal the SGR, but no one is willing to add to the federal deficit to accomplish that. The result is zombie public policy that annually creates anxiety in the provider community and offers another opportunity to heap scorn on Congress for burying its head in the sand.

The indecisiveness over the SGR has cost physicians dearly.

Over the past decade, the cost of providing care has increased five times faster than Medicare reimbursement. Medicare patients require far more complex and time-consuming care for about 60 percent less reimbursement, compared with commercial insurance rates.

Forty-five percent of physicians say they would stop seeing Medicare patients if Congress enacts the Medicare physician rate cuts.

Despite current challenges, 82 percent of respondents said they would be willing to explore new payment and delivery models if a level of stability were restored to the Medicare physician-payment system, according to a Medical Group Management Association (MGMA) survey.

About 60 percent said they have delayed buying new facilities and equipment in the past decade because of the annual SGR uncertainty.

The uncertainty over that looming SGR rate cut was the No. 1 concern for physician practice managers, according to an MGMA survey.

Each time SGR cuts are scheduled for a congressional vote, the nation's physicians become nervous and threaten to pull out of the program. According to the Texas Medical Association (TMA) website: "This decade-long and continued uncertainty is forcing some physicians to make a difficult decision to either opt out of Medicare, limit the number of patients they treat, or retire early. A TMA survey (from August 2011) indicates 50 percent of Texas physicians are considering opting out of the Medicare program altogether."

So far, only about 1 percent of the nation's physicians have opted out of Medicare, according to a Department of Health and Human Services Office of Inspector General (OIG) report. The OIG said it could not determine why these physicians are leaving the program and urged CMS to strengthen its data requirements to track opt-outs.

Who will treat new Medicaid patients?

In many respects, the ACA is selling health-care access that may not exist for many of the newly insured. An increasing number of physicians are choosing to close their practices to Medicaid, which will be expanded significantly in 2014 under the new law.

According to a federal government survey, 96 percent of physicians continue to accept some new patients. Of those who responded, 31 percent said they would not accept new Medicaid patients, 17 percent said they would not take new Medicare patients and 18 percent said they would not take new privately insured patients. The reluctance to accept Medicaid grows as reimbursement gets stingier. For example, Medicaid physicians receive 37 percent of Medicare rates in New Jersey, which is also the state where doctors are least likely to accept Medicare. The average Medicaid reimbursement nationwide is about two-thirds of Medicare's.

In fact, two MIT researchers found that three out of four physicians receive lower reimbursement from Medicaid patients than they do for the uninsured, because the latter have greater ability to pay out of pocket for routine medical expenses.

Under the ACA, CMS will pay primary-care physicians Medicare rates for Medicaid patients in 2013 and 2014. The federal government will pick up the tab for the estimated $11 billion for the enhanced rates. However, this is a mixed blessing for practices, which fear the subsidized rates will cease after two years and then they may be inclined to release the new Medicaid beneficiaries. On the other hand, ACA opponents are concerned that the pay parity will create a new SGR-type political problem when medical groups eventually lobby to extend the enhanced rates.

Medicare payments are about 80 percent of what private health insurance pays, while Medicaid payments were about 58 percent. The gap is even greater between those rates and commercial rates charged by integrated delivery systems with significant market power. Adding to that gap is the fact that Medicare patients have far more complex health-care needs, for which Medicare pays far less than commercial insurance for equivalent service.

Physician fees from Medicaid increased about 15 percent between 2003 and 2008, which was below the general inflation rate. However, Medicaid slightly narrowed the government fee gap because Medicare rates grew even more slowly. Medicaid rates climbed from 69 percent to 72 percent of Medicare during that time.

CHAPTER 3

Health Costs and Family Budgets

To understand the impact of health-care costs on the U.S. household, consider this. The median-income family of four with employer-sponsored health insurance saw its annual income grow from $76,000 in 1999 to $99,000 in 2009. Health-care costs consumed almost all of those gains.

The family was left with $95 a month more to spend on expenses other than health care. If the growth of health-care costs had mirrored the Consumer Price Index, the family would have had $545 more a month to spend on other expenses.

That same mythical family of four paid more than $9,100 out of pocket for medical expenses in 2012, which was 6.5 percent higher than the previous year—a rate that far exceeded wage increases, according to Milliman Medical Index. In less than a decade, the annual health-care costs of a typical family have more than doubled, to $19,400. That was the price of a 2011 Hyundai Sonata.

Families are shouldering a greater share of employer-sponsored health insurance. The median-income family of four pays about 41 percent of the actual cost of health care, a proportion that has been creeping up annually. Employers pay the rest. However, a more realistic view is that employees pay for all of it because most wage-and-benefit increases go toward health-insurance costs.

Many health-reform advocates believe the Affordable Care Act (ACA) will ease this financial burden for families and individuals. However, more than one out of three who gained insurance through the Connector, the Massachusetts version of a health-care exchange, reported difficulty paying medical bills, and nearly half said costs were higher than they expected.

Each household has a different financial pressure point. The media often focus on catastrophic costs inflicted on people with no insurance. The broader story of health-care costs is about financial strain spread across a wide swath of American households. The pain affects much of the middle class and some of the upper middle class as well, including those with employer-sponsored insurance.

Americans actually pay a far lower share of health expenses than they used to. The main purpose of health insurance historically was to cover catastrophic episodes. Before the introduction of Medicare and Medicaid in 1965, patients paid more than half the cost of care out of pocket. That shrank to 15 percent in 2008. Meanwhile, private health plans' share of the bill rose from 21 to 35 percent and government's portion doubled, to 50 percent. The perception that medical bills are the responsibility of someone other than the patient has been a prime contributor to health-care demand over the past four decades.

Despite steeper out-of-pocket costs, the 2011 consumer share of national health spending fell to its lowest level in decades.

Eventually, that trend is likely to reverse. The consumer-share declines have been getting smaller, and high-deductible health plans (HDHPs) are experiencing meteoric growth. Federal health spending also has risen more than three times as fast as consumer health spending since 2007, which is unlikely to continue.

A Deloitte study estimates that consumers pay an additional 15 percent out of pocket on personal health that is not captured by government statistics. These costs include unpaid care giving, over-the-counter medications, and complementary and alternative medical care not covered by insurance.

The inability to pay medical bills and buy prescription drugs is the most persistent household finance problem, according to a recent *Consumer Reports* poll. About 40 percent of Americans had trouble paying medical bills in 2010, up from 34 percent in 2005. More than one-quarter of insured households reported problems with medical debt.

Self-rationing is rampant

Even more disturbing is widespread self-rationing. Nearly six out of 10 adults said they delayed at least some care because of cost. About 40 percent of those in fair or poor health did not fill at least one prescription in the previous year. People with chronic conditions who fail to take medication are flirting with disastrous consequences.

Americans generally cite lack of access as the greatest obstacle to health care, followed by costs. Lack of access can mean several things. In some instances, people cannot see a physician or specialist promptly. Nearly 60 percent say they cannot find care after physician office hours and 30 percent cannot get a timely office appointment.

Increasingly, though, lack of health-care access means not being able to afford it.

According to an ongoing household survey, the incidence of delaying needed care rose sharply between 2003 and 2007. Insured people are among those facing cost pressures. They are paying more out of pocket for care, finding fewer doctors who accept their insurance and facing more limits on what insurance will cover. During those four years, the percentage of those with unmet medical needs increased more among the insured than the uninsured.

Analysts differ on the point where health-care costs are considered burdensome. The Center for Studying Health System Change found that financial pressures increase significantly after out-of-pocket spending exceeds 2.5 percent of household income. Unlike a mortgage, groceries and utilities, medical costs are often unexpected. High medical expenses generally are urgent and associated with serious conditions. Significant injury or disease also may result in loss of income. Even two-thirds of Americans earning more than $75,000 a year worry about getting or paying for future care.

Women experience greater cost and access problems. More than half of women have trouble getting care, and more than 60 percent under age 65 have difficulty paying medical bills. Women use the health-care system more than men do. They often must make choices between getting care or paying credit card bills, the mortgage or other necessities.

Annals of Family Medicine researchers interviewed 33 insured, chronically ill adults who were applying for financial assistance at a nonprofit foundation to help pay for treatment. People were

FINANCIAL BURDEN TO FAMILIES

Percentage of families with selected financial
burdens of medical care.

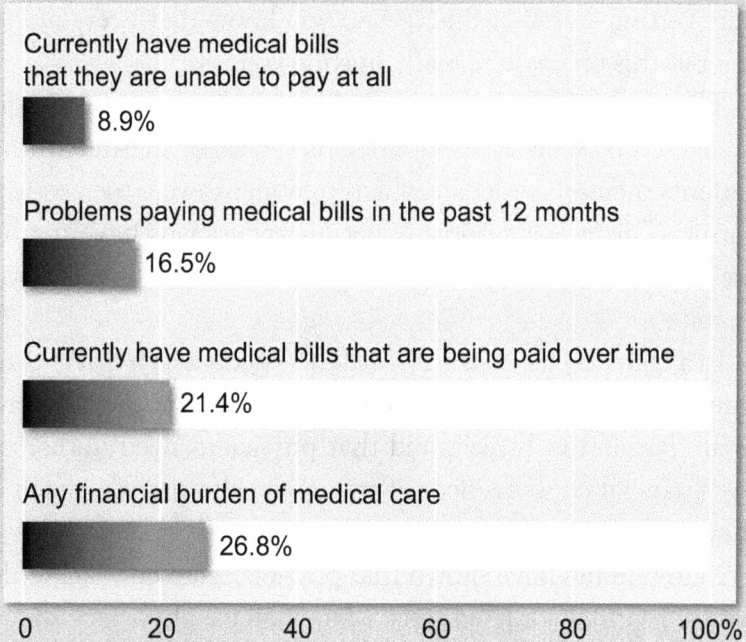

Currently have medical bills
that they are unable to pay at all

8.9%

Problems paying medical bills in the past 12 months

16.5%

Currently have medical bills that are being paid over time

21.4%

Any financial burden of medical care

26.8%

| 0 | 20 | 40 | 60 | 80 | 100% |

Source: National Center for Health Statistics Data Brief, January 2014.

asked about illness-related financial challenges and their impact
on housing, food, utilities, savings and borrowing. Participants
commonly ranked bill-paying priorities, often starting with
housing costs, and described compromises on heating, transportation and food to pay medical expenses.

One participant was prescribed a drug to ease nausea and
vomiting caused by cancer chemotherapy. Insurance paid $900
of the $1,200 cost for a 30-day supply, but he could not afford
the co-payment and went without the medicine. "I said, you

know what, I'd rather be sick," he said.

Another said he "wouldn't go to the doctor unless I just could not stand...the pain. It's scary because when you know you've had colon cancer and your...stool starts changing...then you start getting scared again.... And you know that every month you put this off...you're really hurting yourself."

The study, which also found that people "infrequently discussed costs with their physicians," clearly illustrated that patients themselves decide which treatments were too costly to pursue. This is not surprising because physicians have neither the time nor training to talk to patients about their personal finances.

In a *Journal of the American Medical Association* (JAMA) essay, three physicians argued that "financially toxic" medical expenses are harmful to health, and that physicians need to disclose the financial consequences of treatment alternatives, much as they explain treatment side effects.

Many studies have shown that physicians are unaware of the cost of routinely ordered tests. Many believe physicians should take responsibility for the effect of costs on patients by taking into account the financial impact of prescribed treatment. Others contend that placing this fiduciary mandate on physicians conflicts with their ethical obligation to advocate the best possible treatment for their patients, regardless of cost.

A survey in JAMA found that a majority of physicians agreed that they have some responsibility for controlling health-care costs. However, they believed others had a greater responsibility for restraining costs, including hospitals, insurers, pharmaceutical companies, medical device manufacturers and personal-injury lawyers.

According to the Commonwealth Fund's 2012 Biennial Health Insurance Survey, three out of 10 non-elderly adults were uninsured and 16 percent more were under-insured, meaning that out-of-pocket expenses exceeded 10 percent of income—or deductibles exceeded 5 percent for low-income households.

About half of U.S. households are skimping on other expenses to afford medication, including cutting back on restaurants, entertainment, appliances and electronics, and household luxuries. More than two out of three in fair or poor health care are cutting back on such purchases to pay for drugs.

However, a majority also say medical costs are cutting into basic household necessities, including housing, groceries, fuel and education.

Because so many people live paycheck to paycheck, there has been an inevitable rise in medical debt. About one in 10 insured Californians—and twice that percentage of uninsured—report such indebtedness. About half had debts of less than $2,000, which indicates the number of people who cannot retire those debts with savings.

The U.S. Census Bureau recently introduced a tool that calculated who is poor based on a broader range of living expenses and help that people get from government programs. Using that measure, another 2.5 million Americans are living in poverty—primarily because of out-of-pocket health-care costs.

Bankruptcy: The household nuclear option

Access to care is usually measured nationally by the percentage of Americans who are uninsured. This leaves out people who are under-insured or dealing with burdensome medical debt. The typical benchmark for being under-insured is paying 10 percent or more of household income out of pocket for health care. People under financial strain often forgo needed medical care.

Unlike other expenses, medical costs are difficult to budget for. The uninsured are especially disadvantaged because they receive bills up to 2.5 times what public and private insurers would pay. Unlike individuals, health plans can negotiate lower prices for treatment costs. Only one out of eight uninsured families can pay their hospital bills in full.

Nearly half of the uninsured did not fill at least one prescription in the past year, and more than half had medical problems for which they did not seek care. One out of five had medical debts exceeding $8,000. They lose on average one-third to one-half of their assets to medical expenses when illness strikes. According to a government study, most uninsured people have "virtually no" savings and had median financial assets of just $20.

More than two out of three indebted households say medical spending is a significant contributor to their indebtedness. The out-of-pocket costs driving that debt include emergency department visits, dental expenses, prescription costs and hospitalizations. Nearly half mention the cost of physician visits. More than half say medical bills contributed to their low credit ratings. Medical bills make up the majority of collection actions on credit reports, and most are for less than $250, according to Federal Reserve Board research.

The number of Americans contacted by collection agencies for medical bills rose from 22 million in 2005 to 30 million in 2010.

Medical bills are playing more prominent roles in personal

SELF-RATIONING

Q: In the past 12 months, have you or another member living in your household _____ because of the cost?

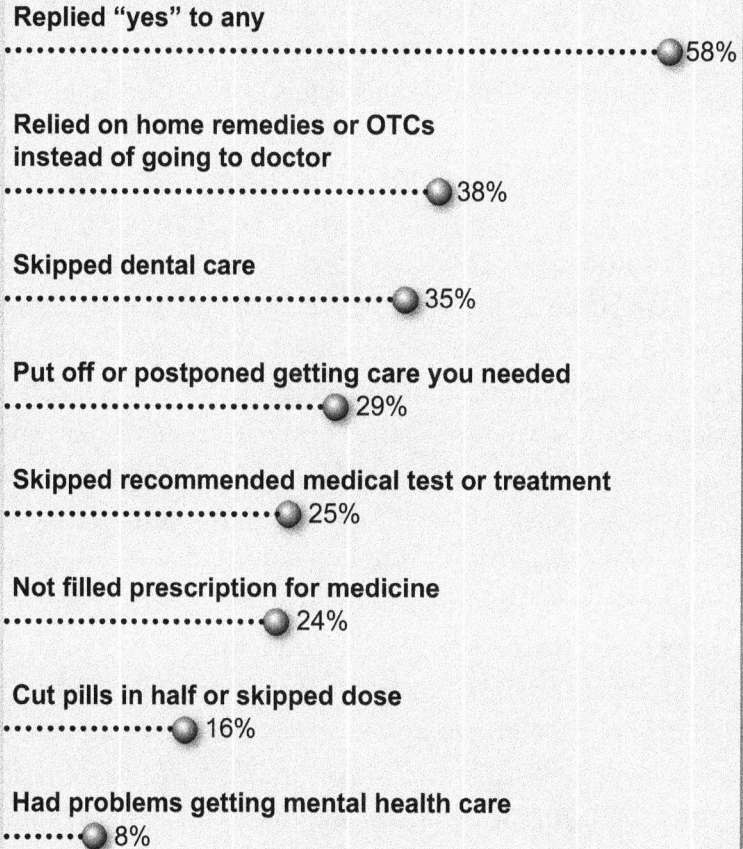

Replied "yes" to any
58%

Relied on home remedies or OTCs instead of going to doctor
38%

Skipped dental care
35%

Put off or postponed getting care you needed
29%

Skipped recommended medical test or treatment
25%

Not filled prescription for medicine
24%

Cut pills in half or skipped dose
16%

Had problems getting mental health care
8%

Source: Kaiser Health Tracking Poll, May 2012.

bankruptcies. Medical expenses contributed to nearly two-thirds of bankruptcies filed in 2007, according to a Harvard study. The share of bankruptcies associated with medical bills increased 50 percent between 2001 and 2007.

The authors were blunt: "The U.S. health-care financing system is broken, and not only for the poor and uninsured. Middle-class families frequently collapse under the strain of a health-care system that treats physical wounds, but often inflicts fiscal ones."

Lead researcher David Himmelstein, who advocates a single-payer system, said in a statement: "Unless you're Warren Buffett, your family is just one serious illness away from bankruptcy. For middle-class Americans, health insurance offers little protection."

Three-quarters of those filing for bankruptcy had medical insurance when they became ill or injured. Many found that they were under-insured and had large out-of-pocket expenses. One-quarter of employers cancel coverage immediately when an employee suffers a disabling illness, and another quarter do so within a year. Medical bankruptcy is rare in developed nations other than the United States. Besides having better medical safety nets, Europeans pay about half as much as Americans do in out-of-pocket expenses.

Some conditions are financially devastating. According to the study, people with multiple sclerosis were billed an average of more than $34,000 out of pocket in 2007. People with diabetes were billed nearly $27,000 and those with serious injuries were charged about $25,000.

Himmelstein also examined the impact of the 2006 Massachusetts health-reform law. The percentage of bankruptcies tied to medical bills changed little after reform, indicating that federal reform will not have much effect on this problem.

Other researchers say such bankruptcy figures are overblown.

They estimate that medical bills contribute to less than 20 percent of bankruptcies and primarily affect those with incomes closer to poverty level.

A study of medical financial burden and mortgage foreclosures found a strong link. Seven of 10 homeowners had a significant medical episode in the two years prior to foreclosure proceedings. More than one-third had outstanding medical bills greater than $2,000, and one out of eight used home equity to pay for care.

Retirement health-care costs

Nearly three out of four Americans who are not retired say they worry about not having enough money to pay for health care in retirement. Those worries appear to be linked in part to the fact that two out of five do not believe Social Security will exist by the time they retire. About half said they are living paycheck to paycheck and therefore cannot save for the future.

People on Medicare are often viewed as being shielded from bankruptcy. Medicare coverage is extensive, but it does not cover everything. A study focusing on the elderly found that medical-related bankruptcy filings for those ages 65 to 74 rose 178 percent between 1991 and 2007—just prior to the beginning of the recent recession.

The elderly have greater medical needs, and their fixed incomes are less capable of absorbing rising medical costs.

Half of Medicare beneficiaries live on less than $23,000 a year, and 45 percent have three or more chronic conditions, according to the Kaiser Family Foundation.

Medicare beneficiaries spent a median of more than $3,100 out of pocket on health expenses in 2007. The top 10 percent spent more than $7,800 of their own money.

Health care is a major retirement expense, and rising at a significantly higher rate than consumer inflation generally. According to Fidelity Investments, health-care expenses for those 65 or older rose more than 4 percent in 2010, compared with 1.1 percent for consumer prices overall and 3.9 percent for U.S. health-care expenditures. Retirees are paying 56 percent more for medical expenses than they did in 2002.

Merrill Lynch investment clients listed rising health-care costs as their No. 1 financial concern in retirement. A majority said they planned to work at least part time after age 65, partially as a hedge against those costs.

The Center for Retirement Research at Boston College estimates that a married couple age 65 will spend $197,000 out of pocket on health care over their remaining life expectancy. The figure rises to $260,000 when nursing care is included.

The good news is that health reform will close the "doughnut hole" in the Medicare Part D prescription drug benefit. Medicare beneficiaries pay out of pocket for medication after the initial coverage limit is met and before catastrophic coverage begins. In 2009, Medicare did not cover the first $295 of prescription expenses, or those incurred between $2,700 and $6,154 annually. The latter gap gradually will close by the end of the decade.

The bad news is that Medicare inevitably will shift more costs to retirees in future years. Retirees spend about 10 percent of their income on health-care expenses. That is expected to rise to 19 percent by 2040.

Working for insurance

The need for health insurance has a firm grip on the U.S. workforce. Three out of four retirees say they worked longer than they otherwise would have, in order to keep health insurance. A majority of the currently employed say they "planned to work longer than you would like in order to continue receiving health insurance through your employer," according to the Employee Benefit Research Institute.

The price of private health insurance has risen five times faster than family incomes since 2003, despite rising deductibles and co-payments.

The average total cost of family health insurance—employer and employees' shares—exceeded $15,000 in 2012, up 62 percent since 2003. Median household income rose only 11 percent during the same period. If the trend continues, family-coverage annual premiums will approach $25,000 by 2020.

The total premium increase does not reflect the full consumer health-expense burden. The average employee paid $3,962 in premiums for a family plan in 2011—up 74 percent from 2003. Deductibles more than doubled in the same period, meaning out-of-pocket costs soared as well.

Large companies increasingly are offering employees only one medical-insurance option: a plan with a high deductible, tied to a health savings account or health reimbursement account.

Two out of three companies with 1,000 employees or more offered at least one such plan in 2013. That is expected to grow to nearly eight out of 10 in 2014. For about 15 percent of companies, an account-based plan was the only option in 2013—double the rate in 2010.

Analysts say the fact that patients are shouldering a larger share of medical costs through higher copays and deductibles will mean fewer will show up in doctors' waiting rooms.

One out of three workers with employer-sponsored insurance —including half of those at small businesses—have deductibles of more than $1,000 for individual coverage. The number of employers offering HDHPs grew by 50 percent from 2010 to 2011.

A classic study by the RAND Corp. between 1971 and 1982 gauged the effects of consumer-directed care. The study divided 2,750 families into four insurance plans. One covered 100 percent of costs. In the other three plans, consumers paid a range of 25 to 95 percent of medical expenses.

Those who were not fully covered spent 20 to 30 percent less than those with full coverage, and there were few health consequences for those who paid more out of pocket. However, consumers paying for care were no more likely to seek out less-expensive care, and tended to skimp equally on needed and unneeded care. The study limitations include the fact that medical care was far less expensive then, and none of the participants was age 65 or older. A more recent study on increased cost sharing among the elderly with supplemental health insurance policies led to an increase in hospitalizations.

In another study, researchers compared more than 200 families with deductibles of between $1,000 and $6,000 annually against 370 families with traditional health plans that had no deductibles. All of the families had at least one child and one member with a chronic condition. The high-deductible families were three to four times more likely to delay or forgo care.

While HDHPs work well for the healthy, they are less useful for those who consume copious amounts of health-care services. In 2009, just 1 percent of the population accounted for more than 21 percent of health-care spending, and 5 percent accounted for about half of total spending.

Another factor that hampers the effectiveness of HDHP plans is the lack of health-care pricing transparency. Consumers do more research when buying automobiles and appliances, primarily because they lack confidence in their ability to shop for health care. Some companies that promote HDHPs offer tools to help their workers become more discerning health-care consumers, but most do not.

Reform boosts high-deductible plans

HDHPs are expected to dominate the health-insurance landscape by the end of the decade.

A RAND Corp. study predicted that half of U.S. workers with employer-sponsored insurance would have HDHPs within a decade, which could reduce annual health-care spending by about $57 billion.

According to a National Business Group on Health survey, large employers now consider HDHPs and wellness initiatives to be more effective at containing costs than making employees pay more of their insurance premiums.

Conservative politicians advocate health policies such as HDHPs that ensure that consumers have "more skin in the game." Traditional health-insurance plans insulate the patient from the true cost of care, they say.

Health reform will take HDHPs to an entirely new level. For those participating in the health-insurance exchanges in 2014, the most popular health plans likely will be HDHPs. According to one estimate, the annual deductible on the plans with the lowest premiums could be $6,530.

Employers increasingly will rely on HDHPs because they want to avoid the law's 40 percent excise tax beginning in 2018 on plans that cost more than $10,200 for an individual and $27,500 for a family. The average deductible for employees enrolled in a preferred provider organization (PPO)—the most popular and comprehensive plan offered by most employers— reached $1,200 in 2010. This certainly blurs the distinction between conventional PPOs and HDHPs.

HDHPs have been growing for individuals and businesses squeezed by enormous annual increases in health-insurance premiums. Each year, the tendency is to gravitate toward skimpier coverage and higher deductibles to maintain affordability. Companies with at least 50 percent of their employees in HDHPs pay about $1,000 less per employee for health benefits.

Nearly 25 percent of working-age adults and about half of individually insured adults have an HDHP.

Effects on physicians and health-care use

Physician visits and prescription drug use dropped among workers who had HDHPs with health savings accounts, according to a *Health Affairs* study.

The study compared health-care costs for two Midwestern companies between 2006 and 2010. One of the companies converted its workforce to a HDHP with a health savings option in January 2007. The other company did not.

Routine cancer screening among those on the HDHP initially fell, and then rebounded by the third year. However, emergency-department visits rose during the third year. Hospitalizations remained the same.

The decline in preventive care suggests that health insurers must "design plans to incentivize primary care and prevention and educate members about what the plan covers," the authors said.

Access to care is hindered either by the inability to afford care or the lack of opportunity for timely care. Regardless of the reason, one out of five Americans had unmet medical needs in 2010, compared with one out of six in 2000.

For several years, the Kaiser Family Foundation has been tracking Americans' health–care utilization. In a 2012 survey, more than one out of three relied on self-help remedies and over-the-counter drops, and cut back dental care.

People with HDHPs generally use less health care. They usually use self-diagnosis, followed by self-rationing. They generally cut back equally on unnecessary and necessary care. Patients tend to give less weight to future health than to present costs.

A 2011 RAND study showed that most HDHP enrollees cut back on care regardless of their income or health.

People on Medicare are especially sensitive to greater cost-sharing, even to increases of just a few dollars. One study of health plans that raised co-payments by less than $10 for physician visits showed a dramatic impact—which ultimately led to more costly care later on. For every 100 people who had to pay more, there were 20 fewer doctor visits, two additional hospitalizations and 13 more days in the hospital the following year. Unlike the younger participants in the 1970s RAND study, Medicare beneficiaries have far more chronic conditions that can flare up without consistent care.

The long-term effects of cutting back are unknown. However, forgone care can lead to greater complications. For example, high cost-sharing causes those with newly diagnosed chronic conditions to delay filling their prescriptions.

Some companies are employing a strategy called value-based insurance design. The format varies the degree of cost-sharing with employees based on the scientific evidence of a drug's or procedure's effectiveness. For example, Pitney Bowes reduced the co-payments for several medications that treat conditions such as diabetes, high blood pressure and asthma. The company's higher pharmacy costs were offset by fewer emergency department visits and avoidable hospitalizations.

A 2007 study concluded that the optimal co-payment for cholesterol-lowering medication was $0 or even negative— meaning patients should be paid to take the drugs, in order to lower overall costs.

Health-insurance companies have enjoyed record profits, because patients are seeking less care than anticipated as premiums and deductibles have continued to rise. It is hard to know whether this is a temporary lull or the new normal in health-care use.

What is puzzling is that HDHPs also prompt patients to cut back on preventive care, even when it is free. This suggests either they did not understand that their policies paid for the services completely, or they are leery of the health-care system generally. They also may fear that the doctor will find something wrong that will result in costly treatment.

HDHPs work well for a significant percentage of the population. However, they will do little to hold down national health costs, because a small percentage of consumers account for a large percentage of those costs. The healthiest 50 percent of Americans each spend about $250 a year on health care.

Treating the sickest 5 percent costs more than $43,000 a year apiece. Even an HDHP would not make a dent in costs for these patients. Once the deductible has been met, the incentive to minimize health-care costs often subsidies.

The harsh reality of HDHPs is that eight out of 10 families earning about $52,000 do not save enough to cover the deductible. More than 40 percent of adults with HDHPs spent 10 percent or more of their income on household medical expenses —a threshold many consider a financial burden on the average family.

Health savings accounts are meant to be an incentive to set aside money to pay for future medical expenses. However, many have difficulty saving for retirement or even vacations—both more pleasant prospects and worthy goals. If people cannot do that, it is unlikely they will save for an unpleasant circumstance such as an unforeseen bout with cancer.

A 2008 consumer survey delivered one of the most depressing commentaries on the American health-care system: People were more concerned about the prospect of paying for the treatment of an illness than about the illness itself.

CHAPTER 4

Passing the Baton

In the public areas and examination rooms of the Southeast Texas Medical Associates (SETMA) offices in Beaumont, there is a poster of a baton being handed off.

The caption reads: "Firmly in the provider's hand, the baton —the care and treatment plan—must be confidently and securely grasped by the patient, if change is to make a difference, 8,760 hours a year."

SETMA chief executive officer Dr. James Holly points out that the health-care provider carries the baton just 0.68 percent of the time while the patient does so the other 99.32 percent of the time.

"Coordination of care between health-care providers is important, but the coordination of the patient's care between the health-care provider and the patient is imperative," he says.

The baton represents the treatment plan. Holly describes the treatment plan as "the engine through which the knowledge and power of the health-care team is transmitted and sustained."

Holly says the baton must be transferred to the patient by

ensuring that she or her caregiver is equipped and empowered to carry out the care plan successfully.

That is the essence of patient engagement.

However, patients are not doing such a great job with that baton.

Consider:

- About seven out of 10 Americans die of chronic disease.
- Nearly two out of three personal bankruptcies involve medical costs.
- More than half of Americans delay medical care because of cost.
- More than half fail to get an annual flu shot.
- Nearly one out of four statin users thought they would be cured after a 30-day prescription.
- Only one out of eight Americans have proficient health literacy.

According to a 2013 Centers for Disease Control survey on lifestyle choices, six out of 10 are overweight; one out of five smoke and fewer than half of them tried to quit in the past year; and one out of three get virtually no exercise.

Physicians can improve their patients' health only if the patients do their part. Physicians need engaged patients to succeed. Too many patients are not holding up their end of the bargain.

Do not smoke. Eat at least five daily servings of fruits and vegetables combined. Drink moderately at most. Exercise at least 30 minutes a day. Sounds easy enough. But only three percent of Americans do all four.

Those who fit the American Heart Association's ideal cardiovascular profile are even rarer. According to University of

Pittsburgh researchers, the profile included seven factors: body mass index of less than 25; untreated cholesterol under 200; blood pressure below 120/80; fasting blood sugar level below 100; exceeds the government-recommended physical activity guidelines; does not smoke; and follows a heart-healthy diet. Of 1,933 people between the ages of 45 and 75, only one person met all seven conditions. Fewer than 10 percent met five or more of the criteria.

The federal government's Healthy People 2010 initiative tracked 733 objectives. Americans had achieved 172 of them— or fewer than one out of four. There was important progress on heart disease since 2000, but obesity and diabetes went in the wrong direction. Rates of smoking and healthy eating rates essentially stayed the same.

Lifestyles of many older Americans have become increasingly unhealthy in the past 20 years. The percentage of those ages 40 to 74 who say they have at least five daily servings of fruits and vegetables combined declined by nearly half. The percentage who worked out 12 times a month was 43 percent, compared with 53 percent in 1988. Even those who had acquired heart disease, high blood pressure or diabetes were no more likely to change their bad habits than those without the conditions.

This age group is the most at risk for developing chronic conditions that can bring premature death or ruin post-retirement quality of life. They often have the knowledge and experience to understand the consequences, and changing behavior is ultimately an individual pursuit. Physicians and pharmaceuticals can only go so far to forestall death and disability. Those 40 to 74 years old who made the necessary changes in middle age cut the risk of death or cardiovascular disease by as much as 40 percent.

Defining patient engagement is elusive. The National eHealth Collaborative surveyed health-care organization leaders about it. Nearly all said it was important. But they could not agree on what it meant.

The most common description was offering patients resources to help them learn about their condition. Other descriptions involved face-to-face communication between physician and patient.

Patient activation and patient engagement are not synonymous. Patient activation encompasses the knowledge, skills and willingness to manage one's own health and care. Patient engagement seeks to increase activation and promote healthy behavior.

One study found that patients with the lowest activation scores cost the health-care system eight percent more in 2010 and 21 percent more in 2011 than patients who had the highest activation levels.

Being a compliant patient would seem to be a relatively easy task. However, a Kaiser Permanente researcher created a chart for a theoretical 67-year-old patient with diabetes, hypertension and high cholesterol and calculated what it would take to heed all medical recommendations. The final tally was more than 3,000 separate behaviors.

Optimism bias

It does not help matters that Americans are in denial about their health. In a poll by *The Atlantic*, nine out of 10 Americans said they were in "very good" or "somewhat good" health. Only 1 percent said they were unsure about their health status.

Yet more than one out of three Americans are obese, and about

PATIENT ENGAGEMENT

Percentage of participants who would ask questions of, discuss preferences with, or express disagreement to their physician when relevant.

Percentage of respondents

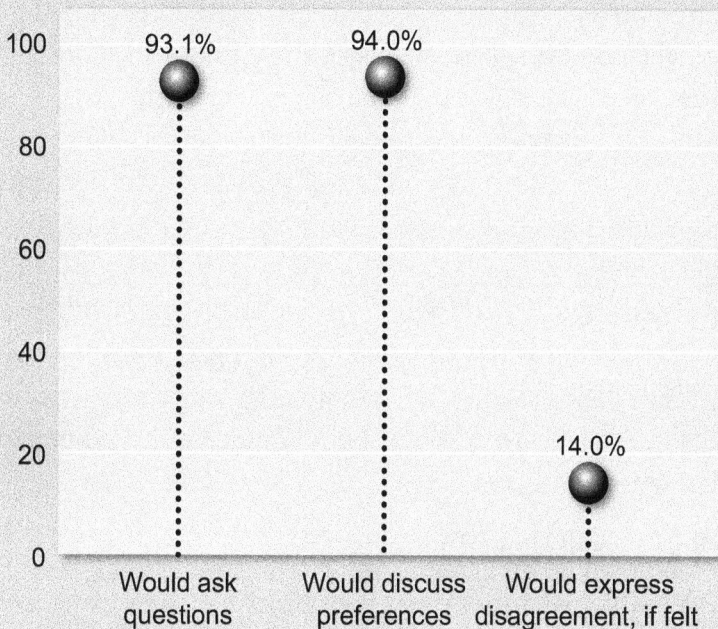

Source: Adams, et al. *JAMA Intern Med.* 2012;172(15)1184.

one out of 10 have a chronic condition such as high blood pressure or diabetes.

Baby boomers are in worse health than their parents were at the same age. They are more obese; have more diabetes, high blood pressure and high cholesterol; get less exercise; and are more likely to use a cane or walker.

A 2009 poll of 2,000 Americans by GE Healthcare, the Cleveland Clinic and Ochsner Health System captured the gap between belief and reality. More than half the respondents said the population's health "was going in the wrong direction," compared with 17 percent who characterized their own health that way.

Only one-quarter to one-third knew their personal basic health numbers—body-mass index, blood pressure, cholesterol, blood glucose level—yet the majority said keeping those numbers in a good range was important to good health.

About 95 percent said regular physician checkups were important, but 70 percent admitted avoiding their doctors by hoping health problems would go away or asking a friend for medical advice.

Pollsters asked respondents to grade their health behaviors, and asked doctors to do the same for their patients. One out of three gave themselves an "A" for nutrition, exercise and personal health management. More than 90 percent graded patients "C" or worse on these.

Physician counseling of patients

Counseling of patients by physicians can have an impact on health behaviors, but it happens infrequently. The average 15-minute doctor-patient encounter does not leave much time for discussion. Doctors also do not think they are very good at it. According to a survey, less than half felt competent prescribing specific diet regimens because they believed they had been inadequately trained.

The lack of reimbursement by insurers for weight-loss counseling and confidence yields predictable results. Only about one-third of obese patients are advised by their doctors to lose weight. That proportion rises to about one-half only if the obesity has created some other medical conditions. Physicians offer to help about one out of four smokers with tobacco-cessation strategies.

Doctors also lack faith that patients will change their habits. Who could blame them? Barely one in 10 diabetics follow dietary guidelines limiting saturated fat. About 18 percent of heart-disease patients continue to smoke, which is not much better than the overall smoking rate.

A doctor's pep talk at the end of the visit does not accomplish much. Success requires a joint action plan and a commitment to follow up. In one study, physicians counseled inactive patients to exercise and had a staff member call two weeks later to monitor progress. Those patients walked five times more than those who were not counseled and monitored.

The American Heart Association advises physicians to use this sort of approach to lower the risk of heart disease. The organization reviewed a decade of research to determine what works best. Joint goal setting, physician feedback and monitoring topped the list. Self-monitoring, such as food diaries, also helps. However, clinical initiatives are employed infrequently because they are time-consuming and insurance companies generally will not pay for them.

Getting past the fat

Anti-obesity campaigns can be thinly veiled messages that stigmatize the intended audience and can backfire. A Georgia public-health campaign bluntly reminded parents that "fat kids become fat adults." A slogan in an Australian campaign: "The more you gain, the more you have to lose."

There is a misguided belief among some that scorn somehow will shame people into losing weight. Ironically, it may make the problem worse. In a study of more than 2,400 overweight women, three out of four said they coped with the stigma against being overweight by defiantly eating more food and refusing to diet.

Examples of weight bias do not get much worse than this: A 2008 bill in the Mississippi House of Representatives would have prohibited restaurants from serving anyone who was obese. Studies consistently show that an anti-fat bias is as pervasive among physicians as it is among the U.S. population.

Physicians agree that it is necessary to treat obesity, but many do not feel competent to do so. Only about half feel qualified to treat adult obesity, and even fewer believe they can address child obesity. About half of primary-care physicians view obese patients as awkward, unattractive and non-compliant, and about one out of three characterize them as weak-willed, sloppy and lazy. About half of doctors acknowledge this bias.

There even is widespread anti-obesity bias among medical students. About one out of three admitted to an explicit bias, and more than half had an implicit bias based on a test that gauged preferences for "fat" or "thin" people. The vast majority of students were unaware of their bias.

Many overweight patients say they are treated disrespectfully by health professionals because of their weight, and more than half of overweight and obese women reported receiving inappropriate comments about weight from their doctors. Obese patients who perceive weight discrimination avoid seeking routine preventive care such as cancer screenings.

In a study of 39 primary-care doctors and 208 of their patients, Johns Hopkins researchers found that physicians built much less rapport with their overweight and obese patients than with their patients of normal weight.

WHERE CONSUMERS SEEK HEALTH INFORMATION

Internet
15.9%
31.1%
32.6%

Books, magazines, newspapers
23.7%
32.9%
18.2%

Friends or relatives
20.0%
30.8%
29.3%

TV or radio
12.0%
15.6%
10.0%

2001
2007
2010

Other
2.2%
5.4%
4.8%

Any source
38.8%
55.5%
50.0%

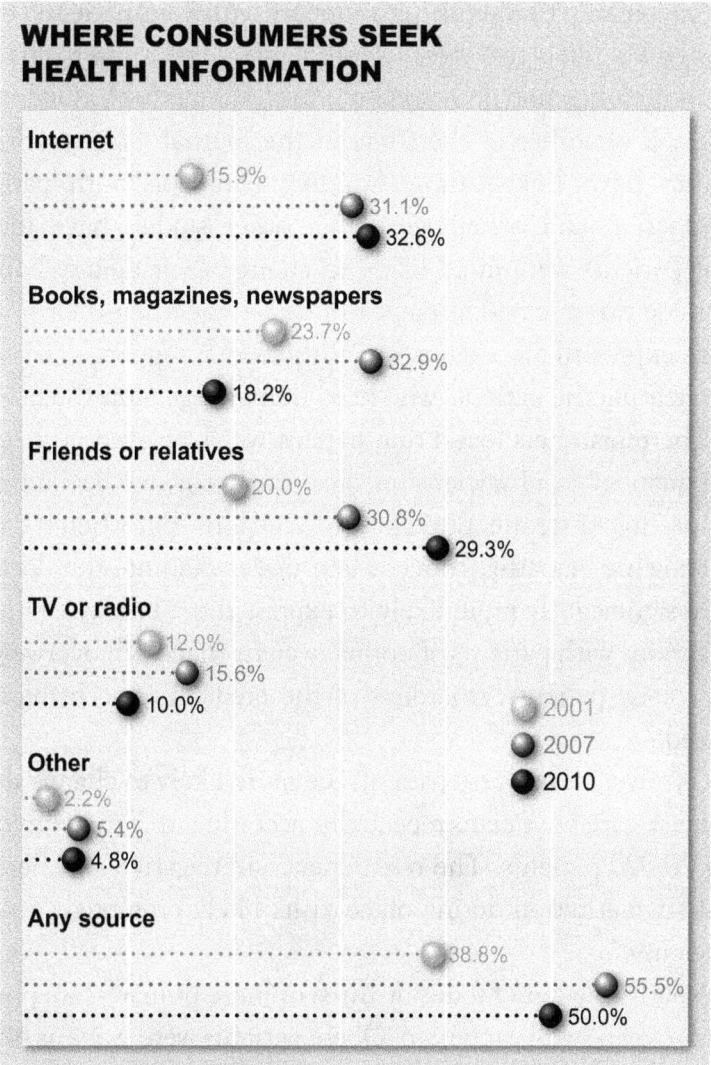

Source: Tu, Center for Studying Health System Change, November 2011.

The percentage of Americans seeking information about a personal health concern declined from 2007 to 2010.

"If you aren't establishing a rapport with your patients, they may be less likely to adhere to your recommendations to change their lifestyles and lose weight," said Kimberly A. Gudzune, M.D., lead author of the study in the journal *Obesity*. "Some studies have linked those bonding behaviors with patient satisfaction and adherence, while other studies have found that patients were more likely to change their dietary habits, increase exercise and attempt to lose weight when their physicians expressed more empathy. Without that rapport, you could be cheating the patients who need that engagement the most."

The researchers found that patient weight played no role in the quantity of physicians' medical questions, medical advice, counseling or treatment regimen discussions. But when it came to showing empathy, concern and understanding, the doctors were significantly more likely to express those behaviors in interactions with patients of normal weight than with overweight and obese patients, regardless of the medical topic being discussed.

Overweight or obese patients are more likely to change their primary-care physicians repeatedly, according to a study involving 20,000 patients. The researchers said negative experiences and stigmatization during office visits likely prompted "doctor shopping."

Nearly one out of four saw three or more primary-care physicians over a two-year period. Obese patients were twice as likely to change doctors repeatedly, compared with those who were merely overweight. Overweight and obese people who repeatedly change physicians were also 85 percent more likely than normal-weight "doctor shoppers" to require a visit to an emergency department (ED). The researchers said many of the ED issues could have been addressed or prevented in a doctor's office and with greater continuity of care.

The impact of a healthy physician

Healthier physicians apparently produce healthier patients. Patients are more likely to follow preventive health practices like getting a flu shot or mammography if their doctors say they do likewise. Researchers found patients whose physicians followed recommended screening or vaccination guidelines were significantly more likely to follow the same healthy practices, compared with patients of non-compliant physicians.

Studies show that healthy physicians are more likely to counsel their patients about the habits they themselves practice. Yet physician health is rarely promoted—despite its positive effects on the healer and patient. Most physician-health programs seem to attempt to mitigate negative health behavior—measuring suitability to practice, mental health, and practice-related psychological motivation and physical stamina.

Researchers reviewed more than two dozen studies on health-care providers' physical activity and related patient counseling. Nearly all showed that physically active health-care providers were significantly more likely to talk to patients about exercise, with some studies indicating that active physicians were two to five times more likely to do so.

U.S. physicians are healthier and have better health habits than nurses and the general adult population, according to a Gallup poll. Physicians are about half as likely to be obese as nurses and other workers, and are far less likely to have chronic conditions such as hypertension and diabetes. Doctors also are five times less likely than the general working population to smoke.

Physicians can lose credibility if they do not appear to be following their own advice. Yale University researchers found that patients are more likely to mistrust physicians and less likely to follow advice their doctors are overweight or obese. They also are more inclined to change doctors.

Change is hard, even for the motivated

Patients find changing health behavior is difficult, especially when there does not seem to be an immediate need to do so. Only half of those given a prescription to help prevent heart disease actually refill their medications. Researchers estimate that lack of medication compliance kills 113,000 annually.

Most people do not die specifically of their bad habits, so it is more convenient to ignore the risks.

Some clinicians rebel against this. An extreme example is a Melbourne, Australia, hospital that refused to perform heart and lung transplants on smokers. Hospital surgeon Greg Snell said it was a waste of taxpayer money to attempt to heal patients who were killing themselves.

"It's about rationing medical resources," Snell said. "There is obviously a morality and ethics base to all of this."

The Australian Medical Association called the policy "unconscionable."

Change is difficult even after life-altering adverse events. At least 40 percent of smokers who survive a heart attack continue to smoke a year later. In a group of more than 1,200 overweight heart-attack survivors, the average weight loss after a year was .2 percent. That is less than a one-pound loss for a 220-pound man.

In another study, 884 of 2,500 heart-attack patients had eaten unhealthy fast food at least once a week one month before the attack. Nearly all received dietary advice before leaving the hospital. Three months later, 503 were still eating fast food at least once a week.

One out of five diagnosed lung-cancer patients continue to smoke. A study of 9,000 cancer survivors found that only one out of 20 were consuming at least five servings of fruits and vegetables daily combined, engaging in regular physical activity and not smoking. However, their physicians do not give cancer survivors much guidance. Fewer than one-third received dietary guidance or exercise advice, and fewer than half had been asked whether they smoked.

Patient engagement: The holy grail

Consultant Leonard Kish likened the effect of patient engagement to that of a blockbuster drug. He cited a 2009 Kaiser study showing that coordinated cardiac care reduced the risk of dying of a cardiac-related cause by 88 percent within the first three months after a heart attack and overall mortality by 76 percent during the same time period.

"Can you imagine what the headlines would be if a new cardiac drug showed this kind of effectiveness?" he wrote.

Kish pointed out that patient and family engagement, which is part of Meaningful Use's (MU) Stage 2, may be the hardest MU goal to achieve.

Better health outcomes and more years of healthy life require patient engagement. An activated patient consistently does what needs to be done to gain the greatest benefit from available health resources.

How many do this? Patients can be divided into thirds. One-third are engaged. Another third are tentative and inconsistent. The final third are disengaged. People with more education, income and self-confidence are more likely to be in the first group. People who do not take charge of their health will fare poorly and be a drag on the performance of their health-care providers under accountable care.

Hospitals will be penalized if they do not provide a high level of patient-centered care. That means they must provide a comfortable, emotionally supportive environment. However, it also means patients will be encouraged to be involved in their own care. They will be asked to participate in decisions about their care and follow treatment plans so they are not readmitted needlessly.

Organized systems of care emerging from health reform, such as accountable care organizations (ACOs) and patient-centered medical homes (PCMHs), will be paid based on the health of their patients. That is a shared responsibility. Access to physicians increasingly will become difficult as the number of insured patients increases. Providers may end up "firing" patients if they are not compliant.

High-deductible health plans will be a central feature of the health-insurance exchanges established by the new law. An increasing number of companies will offer them—in some cases exclusively—as a means of controlling costs. These plans assume that engaged consumers will make wiser personal-health choices to minimize their out-of-pocket costs.

Engaged patients are not deterred by the complexity and fragmentation of the health-care system. They practice good health habits. They manage over-the-counter medications, minor wounds and injuries on their own. They collaborate with their providers and participate in making treatment decisions. They successfully navigate the health-care system, paying attention to provider quality and performance. They seek out reliable information on their own.

Ultimately, personal health requires self-care. Consider that physicians spend about two hours annually with their diabetic patients. Otherwise, those patients log an average of 8,758 hours a year managing the condition on their own.

Research consistently shows that engaged consumers have better health, make better choices and avoid medical errors. Engagement leads to better compliance with treatment, lower health-care costs and better-quality care. Patients do not have the power to change the health-care system. However, they do have the power to change their own care.

The disengaged are overwhelmed. They are less likely to have a usual source of care. They forget 40 to 80 percent of what the physician tells them in the exam room. Six out of 10 with employer-based insurance blame their disengagement on not knowing where to go for information. One in four Medicare beneficiaries are disengaged, and would "rather have someone else tell me what I need to do." One in three of those who are uninsured are simply "not interested."

Researcher Judith Hibbard has developed a way to measure this, called the Patient Activation Measure. The measure includes four stages to becoming a fully competent health-care consumer. She believes activation is constantly changing and subject to a range of flash points that encourage or discourage engagement. She suggests that providers start with the easiest behaviors to instill confidence and break those behaviors down into smaller steps.

The payoff is worth it. Hibbard found that highly activated patients have better care experiences and greater satisfaction than those with lower levels of activation—a critical point under MU rules.

The typical health consumer:

- is able to perform simpler tasks such as making a list of medications, rather than more complex tasks such as participating in treatment decisions.
- seeks out information about a provider or health plan but tends not to use it.
- does not research health information until there is a specific need.
- is quick to cite barriers to care, such as poor health, insufficient knowledge or lack of external support.
- uses the Internet to learn about a condition or symptoms, but it is less clear whether the newly gained knowledge changes behavior.

Shared decision-making

The research on how, or even whether, consumers want to be involved in treatment is mixed, and there is no consensus on a systematic approach. Many are advocating a more formal approach to what is called shared decision-making. The American Medical Association, the American College of Critical Care Medicine and the American Academy of Pediatrics all endorse the model.

Shared decision-making starts with informing patients of the risks and benefits of various treatments or services when there is more than one option. Ideally, the patient carefully considers the alternatives in light of personal preferences and agrees with the physician on a course of action.

Medicine will have to change its traditionally paternalistic culture of care if it is to become more participatory. The patient-doctor encounter as it exists now is not an ideal venue for joint decision-making. The physician and patient have unequal status, and the patient is in a compromised physical and mental state. The physician, under pressure to generate revenue, is in a hurry.

Patients make a large number of medical decisions annually. More than 80 percent of adults over age 40 have made a decision about a surgery, new medication or screening test in the last two years. More than half had to make two or more of these decisions. About one-third of these decisions, in turn, have two or more treatment options. When faced with options, about 70 percent of uninformed patients say that doing what the doctor recommends is important.

When the patients become involved, things change. One study found a 20 to 30 percent reduction in aggressive treatment. This suggests that informed patients are more conservative than their health-care providers are. There are other benefits: better quality of care, increased satisfaction for the patient and provider, and improved self-esteem.

A study of nine common medical decisions, such as whether to have cancer screenings and whether to prescribe medication to alleviate a condition, found that U.S. patients were not well informed. The research also showed that physicians tend to stress the advantages of the treatments they recommend rather than the disadvantages or risks. They also were unlikely to ask patients which course of treatment they would prefer.

The American Heart Association is one of many organizations that want physicians to have ongoing and honest
discussions with patients for shared decision-making. Patients
with advanced heart failure prefer to receive treatment from
their primary-care physicians rather than specialists or hospital-based physicians. However, the AHA acknowledges that
physicians have limited time and training to have extended discussions about patient preferences and personal goals.

One clear barrier to shared decision-making is the fact that
patients fear disagreeing with the physician. More than 1,300
highly educated patients were asked if they could envision asking questions and discussing treatment preferences with their
doctors. Only one out of seven said they would be willing to
disagree verbally with a physician's recommendation. Among
those who would not disagree, about half believed they would
be seen as a difficult patient, and being contrary might interfere
with getting their desired care.

In a *Health Affairs* study, researchers interviewed 48 people in
focus groups about physician-patient encounters. Four themes
emerged: Patients believed they should fall into "socially sanc-
tioned roles" when speaking with their physicians; their doctors
are authoritarian; patients struggle to fill information gaps; and
patients believe they need to bring social support for physician
consultations. Bottom line: Patients worried that challenging
physicians' recommendations would damage their relationships
with their doctors.

Physician-patient discussions should cover the nature of the
intervention, the benefits and risks, alternatives and uncertain-
ties, as well as testing patient understanding and examining
patient preferences. According to a 1999 JAMA study, fewer

than 10 percent of patient encounters met this standard.

Nearly all patients want to play a role in medical decisions. However, they vary widely in how much they want to participate.

- 35 percent want to make the final decision, with physician input.
- 29 percent want complete control.
- 28 percent want equal input from themselves and the physician.
- 7 percent want the physician to decide, with some personal input.

Paging Dr. Google

Dr. Google has been making steady inroads into physician autonomy. More than one out of three Americans say they have gone online to figure out what medical condition they or someone else may have, according to the Pew Research Center.

More than four out of 10 Americans are comfortable using websites that allow them to check health symptoms. About one out of four trust online symptom checkers, mobile apps and home-based vital-sign monitors as much as they trust their doctor. In fact, roughly the same proportion uses these tools instead of going to see the doctor, according to a consumer survey from Royal Philips Electronics.

More than one out of three call the Internet a key to longer life, and one out of 10 said they would "already be dead or severely incapacitated" without web access to health information.

A separate survey underscores the hubris of some patients when it comes to self-diagnosis. Of those who say they "always" or "frequently" turn to the Internet for answers to medical questions, about two out of three say they trust the information, and the same proportion claim to have never misdiagnosed themselves when they rely on the Internet.

One out of two patients worldwide look first to the Internet for health advice. It is a stunning development that half of the world consults a digital device initially when making health decisions. Nearly one in five say they find useful information for making decisions on social-media websites such as Facebook and disease support groups. Only one out of four rely on traditional media—newspapers, magazines and television—for health advice.

In fact, seeking health information is the third most frequent use of the Internet, behind exchanging email and using search engines. Nearly eight out of 10 Internet users do this at least occasionally. Unlike your physician, the information is there 24/7. Women are voracious consumers of online health information, especially if they have children or are conducting research for family members or friends.

Avid users have a nickname: cyberchondriacs. They troll the Web for information six times a month. One out of three Americans did that in 2010, up from one in five in 2009. Most of the top 20 health websites in the world are U.S.-based.

The most frequent reasons for looking online: medicine information; taking a stab at self-diagnosis; reading about other patients' experiences; and researching hospitals or clinics.

The Internet does have a significant impact on health behavior. More than half who sought information said it changed their approach to personal health, and four out of five said they gained a deeper understanding of a condition or illness.

How trustworthy is the information? It depends. Researchers

reviewed 343 website pages on breast cancer and found inaccuracies on only 18 of the pages—an impressive error rate of about 5 percent. By comparison, websites promoting alternative medicine were 15 times as likely to have false or misleading information as conventional-medicine websites.

Many people have gone from simply reading health information to participating in discussion groups and sharing information. This deeper engagement has been called Health 2.0, which is the use of social media that encourage collaboration among patients, caregivers, medical professionals and other stakeholders.

There also are practical reasons for this online involvement. Consumers facing high insurance deductibles are motivated to take a more active role in their care. A 2009 poll found nearly half of health consumers had changed their behavior because of cost: skimping on medication, postponing care and relying more on home remedies. Even when they want to see a doctor, patients are finding it more difficult to secure appointments promptly.

While the Internet can be useful for research, it can become counterproductive. Dr. Michael Fisch, chairman of the oncology department at the University of Texas MD Anderson Cancer Center in Houston, cautions patients about information overload. He told *The New York Times*: "Just like with medicine, you have to ask yourself what dose you can take. For some people, more information makes them wackier, while others get more relaxed and feel more empowered."

Most U.S. adults still trust off-line sources more for health information. Most consult health professionals, friends or family members for advice, with the Internet playing a supplemental role.

About 70 percent of patients who seek health information online plan to ask their physician about what they found. About 40 percent print out the information to bring to the appointment. Distrust of their doctors is not the motive. They seek out information if they are health-literate, believe their condition is serious or want to exercise personal control over their illness.

However, a 2012 Wolters Kluwer Health survey found that consumers might place too much trust in online health information. Two-thirds of those seeking online information said they trusted the information and believed the research makes them better-informed patients.

In a 2011 survey of physicians by the same company, more than three out of four said lack of time was the top barrier to good doctor-patient communication, while about half cited information overload and misinformed patients. However, only one out of eight said patient access to online medical information impeded quality of care and two out of three said they changed their diagnosis based on online information.

Physicians are required by federal law to give patients a copy of their medical notes upon request. Few ask for them, and physicians do not go out of their way to supply them.

However, when patients were offered online access to the notes, nine out of 10 read them. Of those who did, they were more likely to take their medications as prescribed and have a greater understanding of their medical issues than they did before going online. Physicians who shared their notes said the process strengthened their relationship with patients.

CHAPTER 5

Health Reform's Uncertainty

In the lobby of the American College of Cardiology office in Washington, D.C., is an inscription, etched in marble, that reads: "Quality care through science, education and advocacy."

Cardiologist Rick Snyder, former president of the Dallas County Medical Society (DCMS), says advocacy should come first.

"Most of health care stems from science and education. Advocacy is more important," he contends.

Tom Banning, chief executive officer of the Texas Academy of Family Physicians, agrees.

"With all the changes occurring in health care, it is really a physician's professional—if not ethical and moral—obligation to make sure the interests of their patients are heard by policymakers," he said. "For some physicians, that means running for office. For others, it means providing information on how proposed legislation may affect patients and their practice."

Snyder said he encourages medical students to think beyond the science and education of medicine, and to incorporate advocacy to have an impact.

"We need to be more like lawyers," he said. "Advocacy is part of their DNA."

Snyder said he held a 15-minute health-care briefing for 80 freshman members of Congress after a midterm election.

"It went well until the Q&A session. The first question was, 'What is the difference between Medicare and Medicaid?' The second question was, 'What does SGR stand for?' I thought, 'Oh my gosh, we have a problem here.' We need to make legislators as familiar to us as our own patients (to work collaboratively)," he said.

The American Medical Association backed the Affordable Care Act (ACA), over the objections of many of the nation's physicians.

In 2001, the AMA encouraged physicians to be "advocate(s) for social, economic, educational and political changes that ameliorate suffering and contribute to human well-being."

Yet physicians did not vote as often as lawyers or the general population in 1996 and 2002. About half of Americans vote in those elections, compared with about 42 percent of physicians and nearly two-thirds of lawyers.

Grudgingly, physicians are showing muted optimism over health-care reform, despite the obvious loss of clinical autonomy and compensation.

In Deloitte's 2013 physician survey, 44 percent of doctors said the ACA is a good start to dealing with health-care access and cost problems. Signaling increasing acceptance, only 38 percent of physicians said the reform law is a step in the wrong direction, down from 44 percent from the previous year.

However, two-thirds of physicians gave the ACA a "C," "D"

or "F," with a mean grade of "D," saying the law itself would not improve health-care quality or tame costs.

Younger and prospective physicians are more supportive of the law. Nearly half of those younger than 40 said it was a good start, while about one-third opposed it. A survey of students at 10 U.S. medical schools found that two out of three believed the ACA would expand health-care access. Six out of 10 said they supported the law. Of the 15 percent who believed it should be repealed, one-third of those said the law did not go far enough to reform the health-care system.

Yet a Physicians Foundation survey of physicians under 40 found widespread pessimism about the future of U.S. health care. They pointed to the ACA as the No. 1 reason for that pessimism.

Surveys on health care's future are speculative and somewhat beside the point. They differ in wording and approach. One thing is certain: There is no shortage of uncertainty among physicians about the ACA's impact.

Is it indifference or confusion?

Wilbur Cohen, a high-ranking Lyndon Johnson administration health-policy official and principal architect of the Medicare program, once said that health policy is 10 percent legislation and 90 percent implementation.

The ACA survived several near-death experiences—a Supreme Court challenge, President Obama's tight re-election and the ability of the Democrats to maintain a Senate majority.

To understand the challenge the Obama administration faces in implementing the ACA, consider this: Fewer than six in 10 Americans knew that the Obamacare law still existed—less than six months before the health-insurance exchanges were scheduled to open for business. Seven percent thought the Supreme Court had struck it down, and 12 percent believed Congress had repealed Obamacare.

Such confusion prompted Sen. Max Baucus, D-Mont., to declare the law's implementation "a train wreck." Baucus, a key author of the health legislation, said the "administration's public information campaign on the benefits of the Affordable Care Act deserves a failing grade."

Most Americans have no idea of the new options in the health-care law. According to an Enroll America fall 2012 survey, more than two out of three of those likely to qualify for programs did not know that they did.

Physicians are shying away from talking to their patients about the ACA. Only about half of patients with regular physicians said they had heard from their doctors about the law. Of the physicians who did express opinions to patients, there was a fairly even split of positive, negative and neutral viewpoints.

That silence is unfortunate because physicians and nurses are considered the most trusted sources of information on the ACA, according to a Kaiser Family Foundation poll.

Louis Goodman, Texas Medical Association chief executive officer and president of the Physicians Foundation, said all of the foundation's watch issues are related to each other, but uncertainty over the ACA is the overriding issue.

"Explanations (of the law) have not been clear to doctors or patients. When patients can't get information from (exchange) navigators, they turn to doctors. One of the jobs of the Physicians Foundation is to educate doctors so they can give the most reliable answers," he said.

FUTURE OF HEALTH SYSTEM

Q: Most physicians today are focused on their daily responsibilities and unsure where the health system will be or how they will fit into it three to five years from now. Do you . . .?

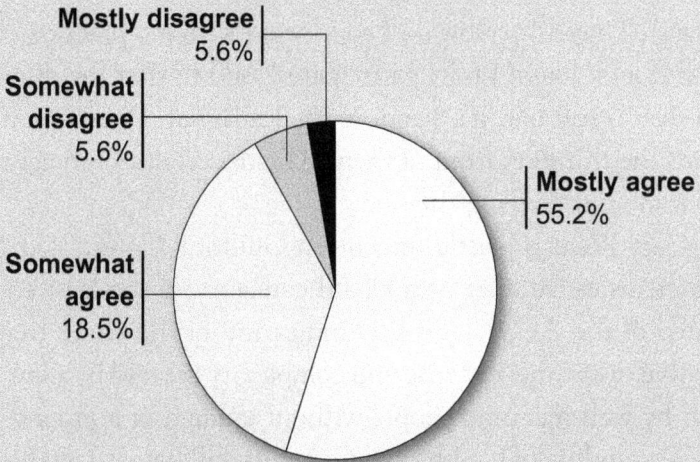

Mostly disagree 5.6%

Somewhat disagree 5.6%

Mostly agree 55.2%

Somewhat agree 18.5%

Source: Physicians Foundation Survey of America's Physicians, 2012.

More than 9 out of 10 physicians are unsure where the health system will be or how they will fit into it three to five years from now.

Goodman said the confusion caused by Healthcare.gov's fumbled roll out placed a burden on patients who thought they had signed up for health insurance on the website, but later learned the insurance company has no record of that patient's sign up.

"It's very complicated. In the 1990s, we had maybe a dozen HMOs. Under the ACA, there are literally thousands of variations of plans," he said.

Claudia Tellez, executive director of the Medical Society of Northern Virginia, said, "Change is never easy. Doctors have the opportunity to be in the driver's seat. They are the ones in control. Many don't see that now. But they will."

Don Alexander, former chief executive officer of the Tennessee Medical Association, said physician resistance to the ACA stems primarily from mistrust of government.

"Doctors still don't have the final regulations (after three years). They ask, 'How do I go forward with my practice? What will it look like if I fully participate?' Add to that the disastrous (website) roll out, it's a case of total mistrust. Doctors can deal with the things in front of them. The uncertainty is heightened now more than ever," he said.

Gary Price, a plastic surgeon in Guilford, Conn., said, "The problems we've seen with Healthcare.gov are the least complicated of the ACA. It's a tiny indication of the chaos that will evolve over time: expense and complexity created by a law written by well-meaning people without enough of a ground-level understanding of health care. Congress will have to modify it in big ways."

Joseph Valenti, an obstetrician and gynecologist from Denton, Texas, said, "The ACA was a deal between the pharmaceutical companies, hospitals, insurers and the government. The AMA was sold a bill of goods that never materialized. In truth, they didn't think through what it would mean to dump 30 million uninsured into the system. Who, and how, are you going to take care of them? You can't dump into them into the Medicaid system and expect them to be taken care of. We'd be closed if we relied on Medicaid."

Philip Schuh, executive vice president and executive director of the Medical Society of the State of New York, said a significant downside to the ACA is UnitedHealthcare's termination of physicians from Medicare Advantage plans because of ACA-mandated funding cuts. The Fairfield County and Hartford County medical associations filed a federal lawsuit challenging the cuts, which terminated nearly 20 percent of the network's physicians in Connecticut.

Schuh also questioned the network adequacy of health-exchange insurance plans. He said many physicians were kept in the dark about whether they were in the exchange networks or how much they would be reimbursed.

Regardless of how successful the ACA turns out to be, Schuh believes a single-payer system is inevitable because employers will not tolerate large premium increases much longer and likely will move employees onto the exchanges or force them into high-deductible plans.

"I think this is the beginning of the end for (employer) health-insurance coverage," he said.

Robert Seligson, chief executive officer of the North Carolina Medical Society, said the ACA "put a bunch of opportunities and challenges into the system. Payment methods will change and the liability climate is going to get better. There is going to be more regulation and more oversight. I am less confident about efforts to eliminate waste and fraud. It tends to get good people out of the system, and the bad guys are too smart to get caught."

More than half of physicians said they were "not at all familiar" with how health-insurance exchanges would affect their business, according to a 2013 LocumTenens.com survey. About two out of three were not familiar with platinum, gold, silver and bronze benefit plans.

Physician practices appear to be rejecting exchange insurance products. According to a Medical Group Management Association

(MGMA) survey, a majority of physician practices believed health-insurance exchanges would have an unfavorable effect on them. Only three out of 10 practices said they would participate as network providers for insurance on the exchange. Of those that said they would not participate, more than half cited administrative and regulatory burdens, concerns about patient collections because of high deductibles, and low reimbursement as their top concerns. More than one out of three physicians said offer rates were lower than Medicare's and nearly one out of five said the rates were lower than Medicaid's.

Providers are especially agitated by a Centers for Medicare and Medicaid Services ruling that gives consumers who qualify for subsidies on the exchanges, and who fail to pay their premiums, a 90-day grace period before their insurer can drop their coverage. In the first 30 days, the insurer must continue to pay incurred claims. However, for subscribers who ultimately fail to pay premiums within 90 days and whose coverage is canceled, payers are not required to pay for claims incurred during the last 60 days of the 90-day period.

"This process unduly burdens physicians, hospitals and other health-care providers who must then collect payment from the patient, and puts them at an unfair and significant risk for providing uncompensated care to patients," Missouri Hospital Association CEO Herb Kuhn and Missouri State Medical Association Executive Vice President Thomas Holloway wrote in an Aug. 12 letter to CMS Administrator Marilyn Tavenner.

> "Physicians, hospitals and other health-care providers cannot reasonably be expected to know or predict if an enrollee's premiums are paid or will be paid before the end of the grace period," the letter continued. "If

the current rules cannot be amended or interpreted in a more equitable manner, we fear there will be a widespread reluctance among physicians and other providers to participate in exchange plans."

Urban Institute researchers contend that physicians will benefit from the ACA because there will be a substantial reduction in the number of patients without health insurance. Nearly 70 percent of U.S. physicians provide low-cost or free care to the uninsured. They also cited the temporary boost in Medicaid fees to match Medicare levels through 2014 for primary-care physicians.

Will doctors step up?

Ezekiel Emanuel, chairman of the department of medical ethics and health policy at the University of Pennsylvania, called physicians the most important group in determining the future of the U.S. health-delivery reform.

"I can sit up here and talk all about it. Other experts can talk about it. Only you can put it into practice," Emanuel said at the annual meeting of the American College of Physicians in San Francisco in April 2013. "You don't do, it ain't gonna happen. It's that simple."

Emanuel said that if physicians take the lead, they can enhance their autonomy and design the delivery system they want, but that would come with financial risk.

"I see no way of getting out of that," he warned. "It's not a dilemma. It's just the inherent nature of what it means to assume autonomy."

Delivery reform began well before the ACA. Patients were demanding greater performance, price transparency and better service. Payers were major forces behind clinical integration and shifting away from fee-for-service incentives and toward greater reliance on information technology.

Two University of Pennsylvania health-care management professors, in a *Harvard Business Review* article, agreed that demands of payers and patients are driving delivery reform. They want health, not health care, and the current system is not designed to deliver that, they said.

They said three "signals" indicate that patients' demands for health will change the business of health care permanently:

- Health is influenced by social determinants, not just biology. "An enormous body of literature supports the view that differences in health are determined as much by the social circumstances that underlie them as by the biologic processes that mediate them."
- Quality data underscore the differences in providers. "In the past there was some implicit presumption that doctors and hospitals provide health care of consistently high quality, that presumption is now being challenged, and we're getting much better at identifying, measuring, reporting and targeting health outcomes."
- Reimbursement is starting to reward coordinated care and outcomes. "Today's standard approach of reimbursing for office visits and hospitalizations is likely to be replaced once better measures of outcomes can provide a substitute that's more relevant to our key goals."

Richard Foster, then Medicare's chief actuary, said in a February 2012 congressional hearing that he was optimistic that providers could improve quality and slow the rise in costs, but was skeptical that they could alter the cost-growth trajectory significantly.

He said: "Many ideas have been developed and tried over the years in an effort to reduce health-care cost growth. Examples include the development of prospective payment systems and other bundled payment mechanisms; the widespread adoption of managed-care plans; efforts to facilitate more prudent use of health-care services through consumer-driven health plans and medical savings accounts; use of 'lean production' techniques by hospitals and other facilities; and, most recently, the development of accountable care organizations (ACOs), patient-centered medical homes (PCMHs), disease management and other efforts to better integrate the delivery of care. Most of these efforts have had some positive impact on lowering the *level* of health-care costs, but there is relatively little evidence that they have succeeded in reducing cost *growth rates.*"

Foster also said that "the prices paid by Medicare for health services (under the ACA productivity adjustment for hospital inpatient services) are very likely to fall increasingly short of the cost of providing services," and that they are on a trajectory to fall even below Medicaid rates.

Medicare payment schedule and pay for performance

Medical practices clearly are leery of new payment models, such as shared savings and bundled payments employed by ACOs and PCMHs. An MGMA-ACMPE survey showed that practices had low expectations about the willingness of large health plans to engage in innovative models. The results reflected providers' frustration at what they viewed as insurers' unwillingness to negotiate and to reimburse adequately for technology and staff investments needed to create the new practice models.

The National Commission on Physician Payment Reform, composed primarily of physicians, concluded in a report that Medicare needed to address inadequate physician payment with "drastic changes" in how it paid providers. The panel concluded there are enough "marginal, harmful, ineffective or unnecessary" services already being paid for by Medicare that requiring more tax dollars would be unnecessary.

The commission urged the elimination of fee-for-service payments by 2020, replaced with a blended payment system based on new delivery and reimbursement models. They offered several recommendations for payment methodologies and discouraged incentives that increase price and utilization.

"The commission concluded that our nation cannot control runaway medical spending without fundamentally changing how physicians are paid, including the inherent incentives built into the current fee-for-service pay system," the report's authors said.

"The way we pay doctors is profoundly flawed," commission co-chairman Dr. Steven Schroeder, a professor of health and health care at the University of California, San Francisco, said in a statement. "We need to move rapidly away from fee-for-service and embrace new ways of paying doctors that encourage cost-effective, high-quality care."

Among the recommendations were increased reimbursement for evaluation and management services; equal pay for the same physician services regardless of specialty or setting; abolition of Medicare's Sustainable Growth Rate (SGR), and improvement of the Relative Value Scale Update Committee, which sets Medicare physician fees.

In a survey of 583 companies representing $103 billion in

annual health spending, respondents said they expected several trends in the next five years: more price transparency; more e-visits and telemedicine; physician pay based more on quality, efficiency and outcomes; and more care delivered through ACOs, PCMHs and other "highly coordinated" models.

Insurers are warming up to new models of paying for care as well.

A survey by HealthEdge, a Massachusetts-based health-care software company, found that more than two out of three health-insurance executives said their organizations planned to participate either in ACOs or pay-for-performance programs in the next three years.

About one out of three insurers are pursuing bundled payments and nearly half are interested in doing so.

More than half said they were giving incentives to members, such as copay or premium reductions, if they adopt healthier habits. There has been plenty of talk about paying bonuses to physicians for keeping patients healthy, but that has been slow in coming.

Primary-care physicians are getting a temporary boost in Medicaid reimbursement. However, government incentives quickly will turn into penalties. Physicians stand to lose up to $1.3 billion a year in Medicare reimbursement if they do not adequately report quality measures to the program, according to an American College of Radiology study.

Although physician involvement in the Centers for Medicare and Medicaid Physician Quality Reporting Program (PQRS) continues to grow, fewer than one out of five physicians qualified for incentive payments.

The shrinking reimbursement could affect hundreds of

thousands of physicians who either do not participate in the program or fail to meet the criteria. Medicare payments will be reduced by 1.5 percent in 2015 and 2 percent in 2016 and beyond if a physician does not meet the PQRS reporting requirements. The 2015 penalty will be based on 2013 reporting.

Another threat is the Independent Payment Advisory Board (IPAB), the panel that is seemingly hated by both Republicans and Democrats—and especially by providers whose incomes the board could put at risk. It was created by the ACA.

More than 500 health-care organizations sent a joint letter to Congress urging its abolition.

"We all share the conviction that the IPAB will not only severely limit Medicare beneficiaries' access to care but also increase health-care costs that are shifted onto employers and working men and women in the private sector," said executives from provider, employer, insurers and other groups in a letter from the Healthcare Leadership Council.

Reform "shouldn't be to arbitrarily cut Medicare spending but rather to achieve better care and improved health outcomes. IPAB is not a mechanism geared to do that," Healthcare Leadership Council President Mary R. Grealy said in a statement.

The appointed 15-person IPAB will have the authority to recommend Medicare spending cuts, which the organizations said would probably take the form of reduced reimbursements to providers.

The recommendations can only affect providers—excluding hospitals—before 2020. IPAB cannot recommend changes in premiums, benefits or eligibility. Taxes and any actions that could be viewed as rationing are forbidden. Payment changes to providers, however, are not prohibited. That puts a target on physicians' backs.

The outlook for fee-for-service

Regardless of all the payment reform talk, fee-for-service is not going away soon.

Only 11 percent of commercial health-care payments to doctors and hospitals is tied to performance or designed to cut waste, according to a new National Scorecard on Payment Reform by Catalyst for Payment Reform (CPR). That means 89 percent of payments are made on the traditional fee-for-service basis, without quality or other performance components.

Among payments tied to value, just 60 percent involve providers' taking on a share of the risk, meaning they stand to lose money if they do not meet certain quality and efficiency measures or if they exceed a budget. The rest are in programs such as pay-for-performance, which offer incentives for providing high-quality care, but do little to discourage overuse or inappropriate care.

CPR, an employer-founded nonprofit focused on creating greater value in health care, is aiming to have at least 20 percent of health-care payments be value-oriented by 2020. However, UnitedHealthcare says as much as 60 percent of its business could be value-based by 2022.

The risk of compensation exposure is tied to what roles physicians occupy in the health-care system. About 50 percent of surveyed medical directors say their compensation is tied to patient stays, safety and satisfaction, according to the MGMA, while only 4 percent of physician pay is linked to quality metrics.

Value-based purchasing (VBP) links information on the quality of health care, including patient outcomes and health status, with financial data. It focuses on managing the use of the health-care system to reduce inappropriate care by rewarding the best-quality providers.

A UnitedHealth Group report estimates payment reform could save anywhere from $200 billion to $600 billion over 10 years. However, physicians clearly are not on board.

According to a Harris Interactive survey, six out of 10 physicians believe the fee-for-service system encourages them to deliver "an appropriate amount of care" and that capitation puts too much risk on the provider. Only about one out of three believe fee-for-service encourages excessive or expensive care.

Physician engagement is critical in the process. However, nine out of 10 physicians say their greatest financial concerns about VBP are receiving inadequate reimbursement and being penalized for circumstances out of their control.

According to an MGMA survey, physician practice executives said working with payers to implement new payment models was an intense challenge in 2013. That concern ranked only behind rising practice expenses.

Most practices said they wanted to explore new Medicare payment models, but were reluctant to do so because of the ever-present threat of the SGR cuts.

The whole concept of pay-for-performance incentives has been called into question. There is some evidence that such incentives reduce creativity and motivation in tasks as complex as practicing medicine, and that they may redirect attention away from tasks that are not being measured. A Robert Wood Johnson Foundation essay argued that pay-for-performance schemes need to capitalize on the inherent desire by most physicians to provide excellent care while striving for a mastery of skills, professional purpose and autonomy.

A Cochrane Collaboration review of studies found no evidence that pay-for-performance financial incentives improved patient outcomes or quality of primary care.

Remarkably, about one out of four physicians said they did not know whether they were participating in any pay-for-performance programs.

Health-care executives sense the obvious resistance.

Paul R. Goldberg, CFO of Jersey City, N.J.-based Liberty-Health: "The medical staff is always the hard part of the process. Doctors aren't seeing anything (economic) on their side related to this (VBP)."

Peter J. Holden, president and CEO of Jordan Hospital in Plymouth, Mass.: "I told (the physicians) front and center that if you don't learn and you don't embrace and you don't exert influence on what's coming, you could be one class away from painting houses."

John Hensing, Phoenix-based Banner Health's executive vice president and chief medical officer, said that a physician's age often influences his or her reaction to VBP. "If you're 60 years old, ride it out. If you're 50 years old, fight it. If you're in your early 40s, you say, 'What does the future hold for me, and what am I going to do about it?' And if you're just starting out, you may say, 'That's the way things have always been.'"

Accountable-care organizations blossoming

Payers are eager to put health care on a budget.

ACOs are groups of doctors, hospitals, and other health-care providers that come together voluntarily to give coordinated, high-quality care to the Medicare patients they serve. Coordinated care helps ensure that patients, especially the chronically ill, get the right care at the right time, with the goal of avoiding unnecessary duplication of services and preventing medical errors. When an ACO succeeds in both delivering high-quality care and spending health-care dollars more wisely, it shares in the savings it achieves for the Medicare program.

ACOs spread swiftly. In spring 2013, 52 percent of U.S. patients lived in primary-care service areas served by ACOs, compared with 45 percent just six months earlier. About 30 percent lived in areas served by two or more ACOs, which was double the rate six months earlier.

However, ACO expansion seems to have lost some steam. After the Centers for Medicare and Medicaid Services announced 106 new Medicare ACOs in January 2013 alone, only 35 new commercial ACOs were announced in the subsequent 10 months.

David Muhlestein of Leavitt Partners, which tracks ACO formation, said there were several reasons for the slowdown. He said there is a lack of widespread acceptance of the model by commercial insurers, and there is no clear model for success. He said many organizations are waiting to see if ACOs renew their contracts with commercial payers, which would signal whether they are succeeding.

Nonetheless, ACOs are expected to be the most prevalent value-based model for health plans, according to Availity Health Information Network.

The report surveyed respondents on their strategy for adopting value-based models such as ACOs, PCMHs, payment-for-coordination, pay-for-performance for physicians and hospitals, and bundled payments. Nearly nine out of 10 health-plan executives said they either had implemented or were planning to implement an ACO in the next 12 to 18 months. They also planned to automate information exchange with physicians in the same time period to implement or expand VBP.

More than half of physicians say they are skittish about entering into Medicare-based ACO agreements with the ever-looming SGR, according to a survey by MGMA. However, most said they would be much more likely—or somewhat more likely—to consider new payment models if Congress passed legislation that would stabilize Medicare reimbursement for five years.

Nearly two out of three physicians surveyed by athenahealth and physician social website Sermo said the shift to ACOs would diminish quality of care, and that such quality generally will deteriorate over the next five years.

Physicians who said they were willing to participate preferred a pay-for-performance model to bundled payments and shared savings agreements. Of the specialties, nearly three out of four anesthesiologists said they were willing to participate, compared with less than half of emergency-medicine physicians. Pay-for-performance is an umbrella term for financial incentives to improve quality and efficiency of care and patient outcomes.

The number of physicians participating in ACOs or planning to do so has tripled between 2012 and 2013, according to Medscape's 2013 Physician Compensation Report.

In 2012, 8 percent of the nation's physicians were either in an ACO or planned to be in one within the year, according to the 2012 survey. This year, 24 percent of respondents are in an ACO or plan to join one within the year.

About four out of 10 physicians are unwilling to participate in an accountable care arrangement, according to a survey by

LocumTenens.com, a physician-staffing firm.

Paul Ginsburg, president of the Washington-based Center for Studying Health System Change, said physician-led ACOs could have more opportunities to create savings in patient care if health insurers cooperate.

"I think physician-led ACOs inherently make markets more competitive because they have an opportunity to shift patients toward higher-value hospitals," Ginsburg said. "It means that a hospital market that might not have large competition going, all of a sudden, if there's a physician-led ACO, those hospitals have to compete on price for the allegiance of those physician-led ACOs."

Ginsburg pointed out that doctor-led ACOs are not compromised financially by reducing hospital admissions and emergency department visits.

Physician-led ACOs dominate

The number of physician-led ACOs has surpassed the number led by hospitals.

Of those choosing to start ACOs, physicians—and specifically independent practice associations—are increasingly taking the lead. The reason is incentives. Physicians can increase their incomes under shared-savings programs. Hospitals lose money when they strive to keep patients healthy and out of the hospital.

Regardless of whether physicians participate in ACOs, they should prepare for the changes ACOs could bring to practice patterns. According to medical publisher DecisionHealth.com, there are five ways ACOs will affect nonparticipating physicians:

- Expect a reduction in referrals at specialty practices.

- Get ready to deal with an ACO if you are a primary-care provider, because many specialists will be part of ACOs.
- Prepare to compete for patients based on customer service, because ACOs will be motivated to keep patients within their networks.
- Play to your strengths if you want to stay unaffiliated. For example, a specialty practice in an under-served area likely would be courted by an ACO and receive referrals even if it does not become part of the network.
- Maybe you should stay independent if you are an older physician near retirement and you have enough long-standing patients to treat.

Despite the proliferation of ACOs, many remain skeptical that they will succeed. Weill Cornell Medical College professors Dr. Douglas Noble and Dr. Lawrence Casalino argued in a *JAMA* commentary that saying ACOs improve "population health" ignores the fact that they can only treat those Medicare beneficiaries attributed to them.

"Population health depends not only on medical care, but also on social services, the public health system and, crucially, on socioeconomic factors, such as housing, education, poverty and nutrition," they wrote. "It will only be possible to have this debate if the phrase 'population health' is used clearly, and not as a vague way of referring to what ACOs are currently doing. Otherwise, it will be very difficult to understand what ACOs are doing, what they are not doing and what they should be doing, who can do these things, how they can be measured and how and for whom incentives should be created."

ACOs that improved diabetes outcomes by as much as 10 percent resulted in almost no cost savings, according to a *Health*

Affairs study. A 4.1 percent drop in adverse events generated only 1.22 percent in savings. Furthermore, ACOs share in only 50 or 60 percent of those savings even if they hit the 2 percent threshold. The improved outcomes also required greater use of prescription drugs, paid for by Medicare Part D and not included in the Shared Savings calculations. Bottom line: Medicare had to spend more to achieve the savings.

That return on investment is paltry, especially considering the estimated ACO startup costs of $1.7 million per organization.

Researchers Lawton Burns and Mark Pauly, writing in *Health Affairs*, expressed the skepticism many feel about ACOs. They said ACOs may have difficulty avoiding the failures of integrated delivery networks during the 1990s, and likely will cost more without delivering higher quality.

They cite the complexity and expense of care coordination and information technology, and the difficulty in recruiting primary-care physicians—the backbone of any ACO effort. They point out that Medicare fee-for-service beneficiaries see an average of two primary-care providers and five specialists across four sites of care. Patients with multiple chronic conditions use even more providers and are less likely to use their assigned physician. Further, a physician treating 257 Medicare patients has to deal with as many as 229 other physicians at 117 care sites. All this seems to make care coordination a pipe dream.

"The path to knowledge begins with having realistic expectations.... We suspect the organizations are not the magic solution," they wrote. "In effect (ACOs) will be told, 'Here is how much money you will get per patient, and you are not allowed to charge any more; do the best you can with that.' This draconian incentive system will truly constitute a test of how much waste there is in the system."

The researchers said the results from the Physician Group Practice Demonstration—a pilot project that predated ACOs—showed that savings came from unmeasured activities such as investments in care management, more intensive diagnostic coding and changes in market conditions. Only six of the 10 organizations in that demonstration program achieved savings.

It is not surprising that many health-care organizations have been shying away from ACOs. A Commonwealth Fund survey found that three out of four hospitals were not considering ACO participation.

Physicians believe ACOs will hit them hard financially. More than half said ACOs would reduce their income while another 12 percent said it would have no effect. Not surprisingly, ACOs report the biggest hurdle they face is physician alignment.

Medical homes more promising

Compared with ACOs, there is a stronger evidence base for PCMHs. These programs, supported by commercial and government insurers, now exist in nearly every state, according to the Washington-based Patient-Centered Primary Care Collaborative.

As of October 2012, Blue Cross Blue Shield affiliates supported four million PCMH patients. Humana medical-home rolls included 70,000 Medicare Advantage and 35,000 commercial members. CMS announced in August 2012 that 500 physician practices, with more than 2,000 physicians, would participate. Aetna, WellPoint and UnitedHealthcare also said their PCMH programs would expand.

A WellPoint pilot project saved the insurer $2.50 to $4.50 for every dollar invested, because of fewer hospitalizations. Patients were satisfied, with about 95 percent saying the practices were well organized.

PCMHs are given significant freedom in how they are organized. Most increase patient access either by having longer office hours or by accepting same-day appointments. Some insurers fund the hiring of case managers or embed them in practices to handle more complex cases. They generally pay practices extra to participate in the program, and offer bonuses for cost savings or quality.

Small practices especially benefit from outside financial support. One study compared 18 practices of one to 10 physicians that received financial incentives and support to attain PCMH status, compared with a control group of 14 practices that did not. After 18 months, 95 percent of the supported practices attained National Committee for Quality Assurance recognition as PCMHs, compared with 21 percent of the control group.

CareFirst Blue Cross Blue Shield, the largest insurer in the Washington, D.C., metropolitan area and sponsor of one of the nation's largest pilot programs, said it created better care and saved nearly $40 million. The program included nearly 80 percent of the metropolitan area's primary-care providers and nearly one million CareFirst enrollees.

However, the research is mixed.

Studies have questioned the impact of PCMHs on quality and costs. An *Annals of Internal Medicine* meta-analysis contended that "current evidence is insufficient to determine effects on clinical and most economic outcomes" of PCMHs.

A 2012 *American Journal of Managed Care* study concluded

FEELINGS ABOUT HEALTH REFORM

Q: How has passage of the Patient Protection and Affordable Care Act affected your feelings about the direction and future of healthcare in America?

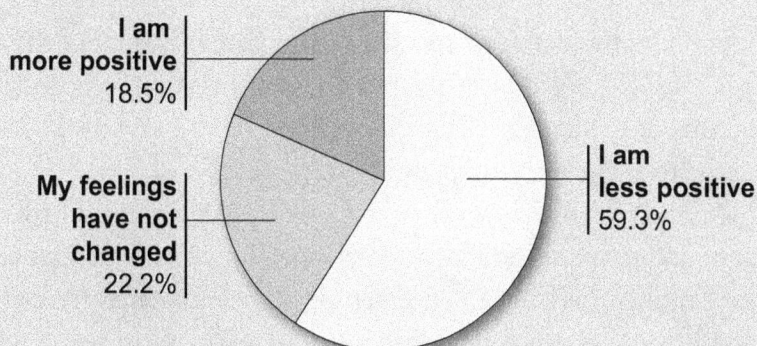

I am more positive 18.5%

My feelings have not changed 22.2%

I am less positive 59.3%

Source: Physicians Foundation Survey of America's Physicians, 2012.

Nearly 6 out of 10 physicians indicate passage of the Patient Protection and Affordable Care Act has made them less positive about the future of health care in America.

that medical homes have some favorable effects, "a few unfavorable effects on costs, and many inconclusive results."

PCMHs can reduce hospitalizations and emergency-department visits because of better care coordination and care managers. However, the savings often are offset by additional bonus payments from payers for the resources to achieve those reductions.

A survey of more than 1,300 PCMH patients found no association between a clinic's use of PCMH processes and patient satisfaction with care.

"One thing to really think hard about in talking about the (PCMH)—this is back-office stuff," lead author Grant Martsolf told *American Medical News.* "It may lead to better care for the patient, but some of these things maybe turn these places into factories.... Potentially, maybe there are these back-office things that make the practice more efficient, but don't make the experience of the patient any better."

From a physician's perspective, a drawback to the PCMH is that most do not benefit financially from preventing hospitalizations or emergency-department visits. Those savings largely accrue to the payers and patients.

Ample research shows that, without outside financial investment and payment reform, attempts to achieve PCMHs can fall short of the desired goals. Conversely, sufficient staffing and equitable reimbursement can lead to greater work satisfaction and less physician burnout.

A federally funded study looked at 19 previously published studies, each of which had a comparison group. The researchers concluded that the PCMH model "holds promise" for improving patient care, but that there was not enough evidence to determine whether it affected clinical outcomes and costs.

The authors admitted their task was "challenging because of a lack of consistent definitions and nomenclature" for medical homes.

The Patient-Centered Primary Care Collaborative criticized the report, saying more current research offered conclusive proof of the model's effectiveness and that "medical-home transformation that requires patience and leadership."

Electronic health records disappoint

The federal government predicted that more than half of doctors' offices and 80 percent of hospitals that accept Medicare or Medicaid would have electronic health records by the end of 2013. Only about 17 percent of physicians used electronic records in 2008.

"We have reached a tipping point in adoption of electronic health records," said Health and Human Services Secretary Kathleen Sebelius, who added that they "are critical to modernizing our health-care system."

Tellez said physicians do not really have a choice about EHR adoption.

"Those who do adjust and participate and engage in health information technology will survive. Those who resist change or choose not to participate, I don't think they will make it (in independent practice). They will become employees or retire," she said.

Despite the fact that nearly half of them had a system in place in 2012, only 9.8 percent of 1,820 primary-care and specialty doctors said they had electronic systems that could satisfy meaningful-use tasks such as tracking referrals or filling prescriptions on line.

The *Annals of Internal Medicine* survey "should be of concern to policymakers," the authors wrote. "Significant progress needs to be made before such systems are believed to be usable by most physicians."

Ross Koppel, a sociologist at the University of Pennsylvania, said in an accompanying commentary that the federal government should establish higher standards for IT vendors.

"What these findings illustrate, unfortunately, is that efforts intended to improve quality and reduce health-care costs instead seem to have stimulated sales and implementations of systems that do not work very well," Koppel wrote. If the systems are to achieve their intended goals, "we must shift from cheering health-information technology implementations to demanding health-information technology utility."

Physician dissatisfaction is increasing. According to one survey, about one out of four physicians were satisfied with their EHR systems in 2012, down from about two out of five in 2011.

Physicians properly adopting EHRs could earn up to $44,000 in Medicare bonuses. However, doctors not meeting requirements by October 2014 stand to be assessed a 1 percent Medicare payment penalty beginning in 2015.

Nearly one out of three physicians with EHR either planned to switch vendors in 2013 or would like to do so, according to a survey of more than 17,000 physicians and other EHR users.

"Meaningful-use incentives created an artificial market for dozens of immature EHR products," said Doug Brown, managing partner of survey sponsor Black Book Rankings.

A separate survey found that nearly half of 300 physician practices buying EHR systems were not first-time purchasers.

The average physician who adopted an EHR lost nearly $44,000 over a five-year period, according to a study in the journal *Health Affairs*. Only about one out of four earned a positive return on investment.

"What our research shows is that a substantial fraction of physicians who adopt these systems don't make the additional changes in the practice that they need to recoup the cost of adoption," said study author Julia Adler-Milstein.

The difference between gain and loss on the conversion was whether physicians used the new system to grow revenue, such as using technological efficiency to grow their patient bases or improving billing.

For many users, EHRs have been a drag on productivity.

A county hospital in Moreno Valley, Calif., noticed that residents were not attending lectures. They were also skipping lunches and even an occasional rotation for the sake of documenting patient encounters in the EHR system their hospital implemented in May 2012.

A resident survey found that switching from paper charts to electronic ones reduced resident productivity by 30 percent, and the average time it took residents to see a patient and chart the visit increased from 21 minutes to 37 minutes.

CHAPTER 6

Relentless Consolidation

In 1994, when Dr. Louis McIntyre joined Westchester Orthopedic Associates in Westchester County, N.Y., the 3,000-square-foot office had nine employees, including four orthopedic surgeons. The following year, the practice spent $500,000 to move into an office that was twice as big to accommodate workers newly hired to handle the clerical demands of managed-care insurance plans, such as insurance verification and pre-authorizations.

In 1995, the practice needed only one employee to verify and authorize treatment. It quickly grew to one employee *for every doctor* to complete those tasks. The annual cost of malpractice insurance for each doctor rose from $40,000 in 1994 to $110,000 in 2010. The practice unsuccessfully tried to negotiate increased insurance reimbursement rates to offset the rising costs. It formed a network of orthopedic surgeons to attempt to improve the economic power of private practices, but was stymied by antitrust laws.

Westchester Orthopedic decided to meet these challenges

head-on with aggressive expansion. It added more physicians and ancillary services to boost revenue. It bought a Magnetic Resonance Imaging (MRI) machine. It spent $500,000 for an electronic medical records (EMR) system. It spent $5 million to build an ambulatory surgery center adjacent to its office.

All told, Westchester Orthopedic spent $6.5 million. It grew revenue from $2 million in 1994 to $5.4 million in 2007, and employed nearly 50 people by that year. The surgeons did this despite the fact that reimbursement rates were falling. The American Academy of Orthopaedic Surgeons (AAOS) estimated that orthopedic surgeons' Medicare reimbursement decreased 28 percent from 1992 to 2007. Commercial insurance reimbursement fell similarly. Then came the American Recovery and Reinvestment Act of 2009, which required an EMR upgrade to satisfy "meaningful use" criteria. The following year brought the Affordable Care Act (ACA), with its quality-reporting requirements and risk-based reimbursement.

In 2012, Westchester Orthopedic threw in the towel and sold its practice to White Plains Hospital. According to the AAOS, hospital employment of orthopedic surgeons tripled from 2004 to 2010.

A study by the Medical Society for the State of New York in 2009 showed that the private practice of medicine was the fifth-largest employer in Westchester County, second among business establishments, third in paying personal income tax, and seventh in paying corporate sales taxes. With the acquisition by a nonprofit hospital, the federal and state corporate and sales taxes paid by Westchester Orthopedic vanished.

McIntyre said, "The combination of decreased reimbursement, increased reporting requirements, the need for huge

MORE PHYSICIANS CHOOSE EMPLOYMENT

Hospitals employed more doctors in 2013 than 2012, and there were fewer solo practitioners.

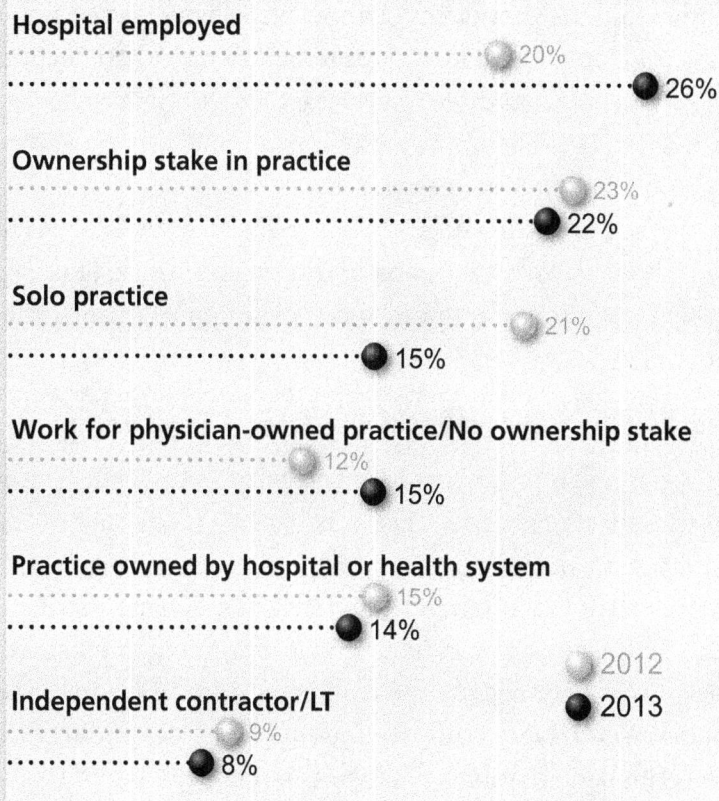

Hospital employed
20%
26%

Ownership stake in practice
23%
22%

Solo practice
21%
15%

Work for physician-owned practice/No ownership stake
12%
15%

Practice owned by hospital or health system
15%
14%

2012
2013

Independent contractor/LT
9%
8%

Source: Jackson Healthcare. *2013 Physician Outlook & Practice Trends.*

outlays for technology improvements and uncertainty about future earning potential is driving private-practice physicians to seek employed positions."

Dallas family physician Darrel Jordan, who closed his practice in July 2012, wrote a letter to his patients saying, "...the changes by the Affordable Care Act (i.e. Obamacare) are designed to add additional stressors and expenses to small doctor practices. This will make small physician offices unlikely to remain open past 2015."

Jordan said the economics of a solo physician practice simply do not work anymore. He said his reimbursement had declined 30 to 40 percent from three to five years ago as practice expenses continued to rise. He said two physicians in neighboring offices were quitting their practices as well.

"I am on the cutting edge of change for all of us (solo physicians)," he said. "We are in one of three stages: those of us who are changing our careers now, those planning to change their careers, or those who are in denial."

'Death by a thousand pinpricks'

Travis Singleton, senior vice president at physician recruiting firm Merritt Hawkins, said it is hard to finger one or two culprits for the declining number of physician practices.

"It's death by a thousand pinpricks. It's the movement to accountable care organizations and patient-centered medical homes. It's the changes in the delivery of care. It's compliance pressures. You have to hire consultants for electronic medical records (implementation). That costs money," he said.

Singleton said the pressures and difficult economics of solo physician practices foreclose that option for medical students, most of whom face large student-loan debts when they are looking for jobs.

"It's easy to say they (medical students) don't want to be a solo practitioner. That's not reality. They may like the autonomy and generational medicine. But they will never have the chance to do it. There are so many challenges facing that delivery model. And that's a shame," he said.

Consider:

- The percentage of U.S. physicians who practice outside a hospital, clinic or large group fell to 39 percent in 2012, down from 57 percent in 2000. Of those who abandoned their independent practice, 87 percent cited the cost of doing business, 61 percent blamed managed care and more than half mentioned electronic health records. Of those who expect to remain independent, one out of three said they plan to turn to a subscription-based care model, such as concierge and direct-pay practices. Accenture, which conducted the survey, predicted that subscription-based models would double annually for the next three years.

- According to a poll by Sermo, a website for physicians, more than one out of four physicians admitted they had been forced to close, or were considering closing, their solo practices. They cited high overhead costs, high malpractice-insurance costs and low reimbursement rates.

- According to QuantiaMD, another website for physicians, more than one out of four primary-care physicians reported poor financial health. Among those feeling financial pressure, 81 percent saw profits fall in 2011 and nearly half had trouble covering costs. Like Jordan, most cited falling reimbursement and the rising costs of practice.

- One out of three physicians say they plan to quit their practice in the next decade, according to a survey by Atlanta-based physician recruiter Jackson Healthcare. Of those who said they plan to quit, a majority cited economic factors and health reform as major reasons.

- More than 75 percent of newly hired physicians will be hospital employees within two years, compared with 11 percent eight years ago, according to Merritt Hawkins. Of its 2,700 searches in 2011 and early 2012, only 2 percent were to fill positions in solo practices, compared with 42 percent in 2004.
- The share of physicians who own their firms dropped from 57 percent in 2000 to 43 percent in 2009, and was expected to fall to 33 percent by 2013, according to Accenture.

An outlier survey by the American Medical Association (AMA) found that more than half of U.S. physicians were self-employed and 60 percent worked in practices wholly owned by physicians. The survey results reflect how AMA defines an independent physician. However, that survey also confirmed increasing hospital employment of physicians. The small, private physician practice is quietly disappearing from the American landscape. Granted, more than 80 percent of physician visits are still at offices with five or fewer physicians. However, there are inexorable trends nibbling away at that piece of Americana.

Gary Price, a plastic surgeon in Guilford, Conn., said health system consolidation would have its most far-reaching effects on physicians.

"The ACA started a tidal wave of consolidation that will never turn back," he said. "We will have single players dominating an entire market. When hospitals buy practices, the cost of stress tests and vasectomies almost double overnight because the hospital simply charges more. The bottom line: The patient sees a dramatic increase in cost for the same service and they are going to be unhappy. We are shifting care from a less expensive model to one that gouges people. The ACA is supposed to

REASONS FOR PHYSICIAN ACQUISITION

Hospitals say they are buying practices because of physician inquiries or competitive positioning.

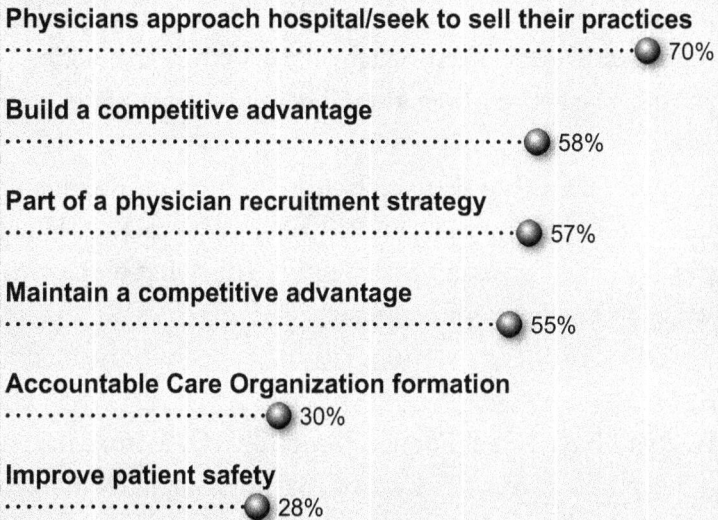

Physicians approach hospital/seek to sell their practices
.... 70%

Build a competitive advantage
.... 58%

Part of a physician recruitment strategy
.... 57%

Maintain a competitive advantage
.... 55%

Accountable Care Organization formation
.... 30%

Improve patient safety
.... 28%

Source: Jackson Healthcare. *Trend Watch: Physician Practice Acquisitions, 2013.*

lower costs, but I'll be shocked if it does."

Philip Schuh, executive vice president and executive director of the Medical Society of the State of New York, said New York health systems are "voraciously" buying physician practices.

"The pace has gone off the charts. Those that are left have no ability to respond and deal properly with government mandates. The future is rather dim for solo and smaller practices," he said. Robert Seligson, chief executive officer of the North Carolina Medical Society, said consolidation "was the exception. Now it is the rule."

Seligson said key drivers of consolidation include delivery-reform uncertainty, declining reimbursement, rising practice overhead and physician administrative burdens.

Todd Atwater, chief executive officer of the South Carolina Medical Association, said consolidation "could be a low-tide, high-tide issue, or it will simply happen. It has leveled off. Those who wanted to have been bought have sold their practices, or maybe we've reached high tide. There are some signs it may reverse."

Atwater said he has seen an increase in interest from medical residents in exploring independent physician practice. He also knows of South Carolina physicians who have left employment to return to independent practice.

Atwater said one of two things would happen in the next five to 10 years.

"We will have large practice groups of 300 doctors and very large hospital systems. Right now, we have about 90 hospitals in South Carolina. ...We will have seven to 12 health systems instead of the 90 hospitals we have now. ...Or we will be five to 10 years closer to a single-payer system," he said.

The aging of the physician workforce

Only one out of four physicians say they plan to continue practicing as they are, while half said they plan to exit the traditional full-time independent private-practice model. One of the demographic imperatives driving this is the fact that one out of four U.S. physicians are 60 or older.

However, more than half of physicians said they changed their retirement plans since the 2007-09 recession. About seven out of 10 of that group said they planned to work longer than they had anticipated because of decimated personal savings.

Conversely, some said they were leaving full-time practice for other reasons: the uncertainty of health reform, the rising cost of doing business or that they simply no longer enjoyed their life's work.

The percentage of physicians in independent practice has been declining by 2 percentage points annually, a reduction that was expected to accelerate to 5 percentage points annually by 2013, according to the AMA. In a 2011 survey of health-care organization executives, 2 out of 3 said they were receiving more employment requests from physicians and they planned to increase their physician hiring over the next three years.

Moreover, third-year medical residents increasingly are by-passing independent physician practices to work as salaried employees in hospitals and larger medical organizations. About half said they were ill prepared to handle the business side of medicine because they received no formal instruction in medical school on how to negotiate contracts or manage reimbursement. It is especially disheartening that three out of 10 third-year medical residents said they would choose another career if they had the opportunity—compared with about one out of 10 in 2008.

Insurance reimbursements are inadequate to cover rising practice expenses. According to the Medical Group Management Association (MGMA), practice expenses per physician have risen more than 50 percent in the past decade, compared with a 28 percent rise in the Consumer Price Index and a 3 percent increase in Medicare reimbursement.

Physicians' search for safe harbor is not the only factor driving consolidation in health care. A weak U.S. economy, capital investment needs and the desire for more market power fueled mergers and acquisitions (M&A).

There were more than 1,000 M&A deals in health care in 2012. That year was one of the most active in the past decade. On the other hand, the aggregate dollar value of those transactions was nearly the lowest in a decade, suggesting that smaller organizations were likelier acquisition targets.

Physician practices were among those with the largest growth in mergers from 2011 to 2012, with transactions valued at $4.4 billion in 2012.

Hospitals traditionally have hired physicians for patient referrals and hospital-based tests and diagnostic imaging. However, health reform has provided incentives for hospitals and physicians to form accountable care organizations (ACOs) and to earn bonuses for efficiency and quality.

The hospital perspective

According to a survey of hospital administrators, 52 percent of hospitals planned to acquire physician practices in 2013, compared with 44 percent that made such purchases in 2012.

The survey found that opportunity, rather than strategy, was the overwhelming reason hospitals are acquiring physician practices. Seventy percent of acquisitions in 2012 began with physicians approaching hospitals to sell their practices.

Even though Moody's Investors Service issued a "negative outlook" on nonprofit hospital finances in early 2013 for the sixth year in a row, it noted that the sector had improved its bottom line in recent years and credited physician-practice acquisition.

Hospitals especially covet increasingly scarce independent primary-care physicians. Dr. Guy Culpepper, president and chief executive officer of Jefferson Physician Group in Dallas has quietly guided his group of about 200 primary-care physicians from the managed-care era of the 1990s to the current wave of consolidation. With primary care in such demand, he and his group constantly fend off suitors.

"They (hospitals) want to buy us, steal us, have us go away and break us up. When hospitals tell our doctors, 'You can make 180 percent of Medicare rates instead of 125 percent,' that is hard to turn down," he said, acknowledging the market power of health systems in negotiating with insurers.

In 2012, for the first time since physician recruiter Merritt Hawkins began its survey in 2002, primary-care physicians generated more annual revenue for their hospitals than did specialists. Primary-care physicians generated an average of more than $1.56 million for their affiliated hospitals, compared with an average of less than $1.43 million for specialists.

"A seismic shift is taking place in medicine, away from specialists and toward primary-care physicians," said Mark Smith, president of Merritt Hawkins. "Primary-care physicians are increasingly employed by hospitals and in new delivery models, such as accountable care organizations. They are taking a greater role in driving both the delivery of care and the flow of health-care dollars."

According to Smith, the volume of services performed by physicians is still the key economic determinant for hospitals, rather than quality of care.

"Hospitals still get higher rewards the more that physicians do for patients within their walls," Smith said. "Volume may not be paramount in the value-based system of the future, but it remains the name of the game today."

The question is whether increased hospital employment of

physicians is a structural workforce change or a passing fad. Hospitals acquired physician practices in droves in the 1990s, only to let them go when it became clear there was a cultural mismatch and the anticipated financial windfall failed to materialize.

Health policy analysts say the current hospital-physician integration will be different. They point out that the ACA is driving delivery transformation, younger physicians are more amenable to employment for work-life balance, and many physicians are feeling the effects of reimbursement cuts. Hospitals need physicians to deliver care and patient referrals. Physicians yearn for income and employment security.

More than half of physicians are now employed by a hospital or integrated delivery system. Over the past decade, there has been a nearly 75 percent increase in the number of physicians employed by hospitals. And hospitals say they plan to continue to step up the pace.

Physicians believe hospital employment should translate into a greater voice in management. More than nine out of 10 believe they should be more involved in executive leadership, serve on boards of directors and have input on performance-improvement initiatives.

There is a history of mistrust between hospital executives and physicians. The former often see the latter as obstacles—rather than partners—in cost-cutting and quality initiatives. The latter frequently see the former as more concerned with the bottom line and their bonuses than patient welfare and physician concerns.

Hospital executives say physician relationships are critical to successful accountable care. Most understand that they will not see a return on investment in physician employment for years, but the improved coordination of care, greater patient satisfaction and larger market share ultimately will pay off.

Acquiring and integrating physician practices are expensive. According to an American College of Physician Executives poll, 32 percent said costs went up after their hospital or health system bought a medical group or practice, compared with 5 percent who said costs decreased.

A Healthcare Financial Management Association (HFMA) survey found physician compensation by hospitals increasingly based on value rather than production. Cost-of-care and efficiency-related incentives are expected to grow from 16 to 67 percent of physician contracts, and quality-related incentives will rise from 65 percent to 86 percent. Care-volume incentives are expected to drop from 77 percent to 59 percent.

Hospitals are just as eager to pursue relationships with independent physicians. Nearly one out of three are pursuing clinical relationships, directorships and co-management opportunities with independent physicians.

Hospital consolidation

Hospitals also are consolidating among themselves. In 2013, more than three out of four either were exploring a possible merger or were in the midst of one.

Hospitals and health systems are consolidating horizontally and vertically. About 60 percent of hospitals are part of health systems, up from 53 percent 10 years ago. The average local system has 3.2 independent hospitals.

According to Harvard economist David Cutler, the top three market-share leaders in an average Medicare hospital-referral region account for more than three out of four hospital admissions. Cutler describes the typical hospital market as one dominant system, two or three smaller systems and a fringe of even smaller institutions.

There has been a steady increase in hospital M&A deals in the past decade. In 2003, there were 38 M&A deals involving 56 hospitals. In 2011, there were 90 deals involving 156 hospitals. From 2007 to 2012, 432 deals were announced, involving 835 hospitals.

HFMA identified three major forces behind recent hospital mergers:

- The need to improve economies of scale and market leverage in negotiations with payers.
- Physician employees, technology and regulatory compliance are raising overhead costs.
- The drive to create accountable care delivery systems to improve quality and lower costs.

One of the biggest recent acquisitions was Tenet Healthcare Corp.'s purchase of Vanguard Health Systems, creating a system of nearly 80 hospitals and twice that many outpatient centers in 16 states.

Tenet CEO Trevor Fetter said in a statement that the company's emerging aggressive buying strategy is necessary "to compete effectively in a rapidly changing environment."

Tenet itself was the target of a contentious and unsuccessful 2011 takeover by Community Health Systems.

Hospital consolidation is reminiscent of the creation of integrated delivery systems in the 1990s.

Jack Hess, a partner at Financial Resource Group in Dallas

and a former hospital executive, said the dominant 1990s strategy was to get bigger to negotiate with managed-care companies, an approach that included acquisition—and often "de-acquisition"—of physician practices.

Jim Berend, a partner at the consulting firm Grant Thornton International in Dallas, said the 1990s were driven more by fear, including fear of managed-care organizations and the strength of for-profit hospital systems. He said many providers believed they could not compete without being large.

Attorney Tom Watson, managing partner at accounting firm BKD in Dallas, said current M&A activity is driven by regulatory issues.

"They are asking: 'Can we survive under this regulatory environment? Am I big enough?'"

Barry Sagraves, managing director at Juniper Advisory in Chicago, said some health systems are "getting bigger for the sake of getting bigger. There is confusion between size and scale. Many are getting bigger without figuring out how to achieve cost savings and quality."

Berend said most of the few remaining independent hospitals are financially strong. However, the effects of Medicare reimbursement cuts may take their toll, and those hospitals may find that sitting on the sidelines no longer works.

Watson said he works with a number of smaller hospitals. He said they are fighting to remain independent because they are significant players in their local economies.

"They don't want to give the car keys to economic development to someone (in a distant city). They want to keep local control and protect a community asset," he said.

Cleveland Clinic President Delos "Toby" Cosgrove told

HealthLeaders Media that health systems increasingly are trying to find linkages in disparate markets to improve efficiencies, rather than striving for market dominance. Health systems are acquiring struggling hospitals and health systems "to turn around their finances and reap the benefits of consolidation," Cosgrove said.

A Robert Wood Johnson Foundation synthesis of hospital studies found that hospital consolidation had led to neither improved quality nor lower costs. The study suggested that the primary purpose of consolidation was to improve bargaining power with commercial payers. When hospitals merged in already-concentrated markets, prices rose by as much as 40 percent. Conversely, the analysis found that hospital competition improved overall quality of care.

The study made a distinction between consolidation and integration. The former simply brings together previously independent entities with minimal operational and personnel changes. The latter eliminates unnecessary duplication, merging separate entities under comprehensive management.

Karen Ignagni, chief executive officer of the trade group America's Health Insurance Plans, told The New York Times, "The rhetoric (of hospital mergers) is all about efficiency. The reality is all about higher prices."

The resulting cost increases have not gone unnoticed. The Federal Trade Commission (FTC) has begun to block some health-care mergers. In February 2013, the Supreme Court confirmed the agency's authority to challenge the merger of two hospitals in Georgia. The following month, the FTC filed a lawsuit to block an Idaho hospital chain's purchase of the largest multi-specialty independent physicians' practice. In 2012, the agency stopped the purchase of a surgical center by a hospital in

Pennsylvania.

By 2006, more than 75 percent of U.S. metropolitan areas already had experienced enough hospital merger activity to be considered "highly consolidated."

Yet apparently more is coming. Consulting firm Booz & Company estimates about 20 percent of U.S. hospitals will have new owners by the end of the decade.

Health reform likely will accelerate hospital consolidation. Consultant PwC examined trends in Massachusetts after the state implemented universal health care in 2007. It found that one out of three of the state's 70 hospitals merged, acquired or partnered with another health system.

According to PwC, Massachusetts community hospitals consolidated with larger systems mainly to improve their financial positions by offsetting costs and maximizing returns on new payment models and referrals. The state's safety-net hospitals sought out financially stronger partners, especially after the state reduced reimbursement for low-income patients and the hospitals faced more cuts under the ACA, according to PwC.

Hospital-physician consolidation

Grant Thornton says hospitals are acquiring physician practices at a more rapid rate because they need a secure physician base amid impending doctor shortages, the need to create new delivery models to meet payer-driven cost and quality initiatives, and general market uncertainty.

After initially knocking the trend, analysts began applauding hospital employment of physicians. According to Fitch Ratings and Moody's Investors Service, physician employment has allowed hospitals to overcome flat inpatient revenue with greater outpatient care. Health reform is driving a shift from inpatient to more cost-effective outpatient sites.

Fitch said the No. 1 health-care sector challenge in 2014 would be to maintain profitability despite weak patient volumes and declining Medicare reimbursement to hospitals.

Moody's partially attributed the gains to physicians. Closer relationships with physicians have helped hospitals stabilize their market shares and cut costs, Moody's said. The relationships have translated into more physician input through joint ventures and hospital board memberships, aided by accelerating physician-practice acquisition. The rating service credited such steps, which ensure a steady flow of patient referrals, as an antidote to hospital reimbursement cuts stemming from the ACA.

According to Moody's, inpatient admissions have been flat or declined since 2009, compared with physician office-visit growth of nearly 5 percent. Hospital profit margins stabilized in 2011 at about 2.5 percent.

A *Wall Street Journal* report noted the effect of physician employment on the cost of care. It pointed out that a 15-minute physician visit might cost about $70 at an independent practice, compared with $124 at a hospital outpatient clinic. Hospitals are able to use their market power to negotiate higher reimbursement rates with commercial payers, and Medicare pays "substantially" more when procedures are performed at a hospital-owned facility.

For Merritt Hawkins, 63 percent of physician searches between April 2011 and March 2012 were for hospitals, compared with 56 percent the year before.

One reason for greater physician demand is that physicians are working fewer hours. Compared with 2008, doctors now are working about 6 percent fewer hours and are seeing nearly 17 percent fewer patients per day, according to the Physicians Foundation.

Looming retirement for aging and frustrated physicians also is a factor. Nearly one out of four physicians are past the age of 60, and many delayed retirement because of the recent recession. Many others want nothing to do with the ACA. The Physicians Foundation survey estimated that 80,000 to 100,000 doctors might retire between 2012 and 2018.

Hospitals are recruiting physicians even when they do not have openings. More than half were recruiting for expected openings and nearly an equal number said they stockpiled candidates.

The percentage of cardiologists who were employed by hospitals tripled from 8 percent in 2007 to 24 percent in 2012, according to an American College of Cardiology survey.

Physicians who become employees increasingly consider themselves free agents, often open to the best opportunity. More than half working for hospital-owned or large independent groups were seeking to change practices for financial security, and a nearly equal number generally were dissatisfied with their current work circumstances.

More than half of practicing physicians get at least three employment solicitations a week. Almost 29 percent receive three to five weekly. Twenty-three percent get six to 10 notices, according to the Medicus Firm, a physician recruiter. Medicus also found that signing bonuses, once considered optional, are now an expectation.

According to a survey by QuantiaMD, an online physician community, about half of employed primary-care physicians had not had a raise in one to two years. Nearly one out of five had experienced a cut in salary.

The AMA House of Delegates approved a set of six principles for physicians who become employees. They included guidelines on peer review, payment agreements and conflicts of interest.

Hospitals and health systems are changing executive compensation to include physician alignment. More than a third used some type of physician alignment criteria in their incentive plans in 2012, according to a survey by consulting firm Integrated Healthcare Strategies.

Increasing use of employment contracts

The use of employment contracts and incentives increased in 2012 for both hospital-based and physician-group practices, according to a survey by The Hay Group, a global management consulting firm.

In hospitals, 70 percent of physicians had employment contracts, compared with 64 percent in 2011. About two out of three physicians in group-based practices had contracts in 2012, compared with 56 percent in 2011.

Incentives largely were determined by quality and patient satisfaction. About 77 percent of organizations reported that they used quality, and 66 percent relied on patient satisfaction, to measure physician performance. Conversely, only 39 percent reported "outcomes" as a performance metric for physicians.

Nearly nine out of 10 organizations provided malpractice insurance to their physicians. Almost all provided the insurance at no cost.

Physician pay increases will rise slightly in 2013, according to

Hay Group's annual physician compensation survey.

Physician turnover is at a record high, according to a survey by Cejka Search and the American Medical Group Association.

Physician turnover in medical groups averaged 6.8 percent in 2012, compared with 6.5 percent in 2011 and 5.9 percent in 2009. More than one out of three physician groups expected the physician retirement rate to increase again in 2013. The survey included 80 physician groups composed of nearly 20,000 physicians.

One measure of that turnover is a spike in demand for nurse practitioners and physician assistants to fill vacant physician positions temporarily. About one out of 10 staffing requests from hospitals and clinics in 2012 were for NPs or PAs, compared with 2 percent in 2010.

Staff Care is a staffing firm that provides temporary physicians and allied health-care professionals to hospitals, medical groups, government facilities and other health-care organizations. Bonnie Owens, Staff Care vice president, said this is the first time in Staff Care's history that the No. 1 reason for seeking part-time providers is the need to fill in for a departing physician. She said that reflected the rapid absorption of physician practices by health systems.

Staff Care estimates the ranks of temporary, or locum tenens, physicians has swelled from 26,000 a decade ago to about 38,000 now.

The employment binge seems quixotic. According to Dr. Robert Kocher, a former Obama administration health-care adviser, hospitals lose $150,000 to $250,000 a year for the first three years they employ a physician as the doctor builds up a patient panel. After that, hospitals expect to make money on employed physicians after accounting for the value of care, tests and referrals.

As American Enterprise Institute's Dr. Scott Gottlieb pointed out in a 2013 *Wall Street Journal* essay, MGMA found that physician productivity drops by more than 25 percent after being employed. Physicians no longer feel bound to work long hours for the sake of a practice's survival.

Steve Corso is MedSynergies' managing director of physician engagement. His job is to align hospitals and physicians as the marketplace consolidates and delivery reform unfolds. He recently wrote a white paper on the subject. He also happens to be the son of ESPN college football analyst and former coach Lee Corso.

Here are some common errors he sees after health systems acquire physician practices:

- **Not managing expectations.** "Physicians don't understand why they are not in control of the changes taking place."
- **Not adjusting system management to accommodate the acquisitions.** "(The new practices) come flying into the bureaucracy, and there has been no preparation. You wake up one day and realize you now have 50 physician practices and 1,000 physicians. Health systems assume you can use hospital-trained staff to manage doctors. The physician enterprise needs its own space and breathing room. This is a merger, and even the best companies have trouble with mergers."
- **Not harnessing physician leadership.** "Put a physician in charge. Don't appoint them. Let the physicians have a

say in who will lead. It helps lower the political drama of change."

- **Lacking clarity of purpose.** "It's like a sports team. The Los Angeles Lakers have great players. If there is no unity of purpose, you can have individuals making great individual plays, but not a great team. Primary care has to meet cardiology. You have to ask, 'How can we make ourselves better and win market share?'"

- **Not engaging physicians individually about their changed circumstances.** "Doctors say, 'I don't know how I fit into this system. I don't understand my personal impact.' You have to give them a vision of the value proposition, how they fit in personally. They need to understand how and why things are changing, and that it is in their best interest to embrace that change. They may not completely agree, but they understand."

Corso has advice for physicians as well.

"Being the squeaky wheel worked under the old model. It does not work so well once you are employed. Becoming an influencer works much better," he said.

Corso foresees a future where systems engage physicians constantly, from courtship to acquisition to assimilation. He said systems increasingly will build it into hospital-executive compensation and there will be better tools to measure it.

"Alignment isn't just a word. It takes a lot of work and has many touch points. It will grow as a discipline," he said.

Insurers getting into the act

Like hospitals and health systems, health insurers believe that getting bigger will give them an advantage in the post-health-reform marketplace. They expect to continue to consolidate.

That could be a problem for independent physicians. Greater insurer market power could mean even less leverage in fee negotiations and pressure to participate in health plans' Medicaid managed care and Medicare Advantage networks.

One health insurer has a market share of 50 percent or more in the individual market in 30 states, according to a 2011 Kaiser Family Foundation study. A similar 2012 analysis by the American Medical Association found a lack of health insurer competition in 70 percent of the nation's metropolitan areas, and that two insurers had a commercial market share of 50 percent or more in 45 states. Physicians charge that such concentration creates higher premiums, skimpier health benefits for consumers and lower physician reimbursement.

Insurers also are diversifying into patient care. Four of the five largest health insurers increased their physician holdings in the past year, and some are launching practice management companies.

Some see this as an effort by payers to create a countervailing force against hospital-led ACOs. They see it as a strategic maneuver in the market-by-market negotiating battles waged by insurance companies and large health-care organizations.

During the heyday of managed care in the 1990s, insurers were seen as bullies attempting to impose cost control and utilization muscle. The effort buckled after enormous push back by providers and patients. Insurers are now trying to be part of the solution by assisting providers who want to deliver high-quality, cost-effective care.

Although patient-centered medical homes are associated with health reform and Medicare innovations, health insurance companies are rolling out pilot projects for working-age adults. They are finding that paying incentives to primary-care physicians to keep patients away from the hospital and high-cost specialists is a winning business model.

About one-third of health-care dollars are spent on hospital care, and about 20 percent are spent on physician services and specialists.

CHAPTER 7

Triaging the Newly Insured

A group of Medical University of South Carolina (MUSC) students solemnly surrounds a dummy patient in a simulated emergency-department (ED) treatment room. The attending team includes a senior medical student, two third-year pharmacy students, a second-year nursing student and a first-year physician assistant. The simulation is being filmed for later debriefing with the professor.

The clinicians interview the lifeless mass of rubber, probing for symptoms and treatment history. A disembodied voice—supplied by a faculty member in another room—answers the questions over loudspeakers.

The "patient" is a 59-year-old woman who complains of lethargy, nausea and a dry cough that has gotten worse over two days. She is also concerned about "some mild chest pain." She denies fever, palpitations and syncope. She was admitted to the hospital for pneumonia last week and hospitalized for three days. She was discharged to home two days ago.

The team consults as it works. One of the team members

writes treatment orders on a white board.

Dr. Donna Kern, assistant dean for patient safety and simulation, looks on from a video monitor. "What we look for," she says, "is whether the team leader—the doctor—is a good communicator and uses team members."

Kern likes the physician in this simulation because he delegates tasks to his team members. She also likes the fact that he admits to the patient that the reason she has returned to the ED is that she was prescribed the wrong medication. He apologizes to the patient for the error, even though he did not make the mistake.

Kern, who is a stickler for error disclosure, says, "He is the only one (this semester) who apologized. Only two out of the 24 teams (evaluated) explained the error. It's amazing how, even without training, students start spinning and word smithing rather than be transparent."

MUSC has become a leader in what is called inter-professional education (IPE). Students are taught team-based care, to the point that it is part of the school's instructional DNA. MUSC packs six colleges, more than 3,000 students and medical residents, and 1,500 faculty members into four city blocks. The schools—medicine, nursing, pharmacy, health professions, dental and biomedicine—share centralized classrooms. The university operates a 750-bed medical center and has a combined annual budget of $1.7 billion.

Three nights a week, students see uninsured patients in MUSC's 1,000-square-foot medical clinic in Mount Pleasant, northeast of Charleston Harbor. A team of up to three students meets with patients on a first-come, first-serve basis. The team interviews patients in the clinic's two exam rooms and then huddles with an attending physician to present the cases before diagnosing conditions and prescribing treatments. The students' caseload is largely preventive and primary care.

Students are responsible for the management of the clinic, called the Community Aid, Relief, Education and Support Clinic (CARES). During a calendar year, students volunteer more than 5,000 hours of labor to treat nearly 2,000 patients.

Dr. Wanda Gonsalves, associate professor of family medicine and medical director of MUSC's physician assistant program, is the faculty supervisor. She was involved in a similar free clinic when she was at the University of Kentucky.

She calls the clinic "the quintessential IPE experience." Teams combine first- or second-year medical students with a third- or fourth-year student. Other team members include a physician assistant and a pharmacy student. She said students "learn the value of everyone else" on the team.

The Association of American Medical Colleges (AAMC) encourages IPE. That style of teaching is more common in the United Kingdom and Canada, although it is increasingly common in the U.S. Inter-professional training either is under way or being developed at East Tennessee State University, the University of California at San Diego, Loyola University Chicago, the University of Kentucky and Thomas Jefferson University in Philadelphia.

Dr. Carol Aschenbrener, AAMC's chief medical education officer, told *American Medical News,* "Every health professional needs to be prepared for collaborative practice. The needs of the population are more complex and can't be met by any one profession."

Team-based care has become the foundation of patient-

centered medical homes (PCMH) and accountable care organizations, and is the most-proffered solution for the widening
physician shortage. Even if it is a solution, the question remains
whether the culture of physician practices will change quickly
enough to embrace team care to treat the newly insured and an
aging population.

The MUSC model is in stark contrast to the traditional
health-care education strategy: keep members of different professions separate until they are fully trained, and then attempt
to get them to work together. This approach often ingrains atti-
tudinal biases, lack of understanding of others' professional roles
and expertise, and an absence of team-building skills.

The federal government's effort to address the nation's
health-care workforce fits its do-nothing caricature.

The National Health Care Workforce Commission was
charged with helping prepare the nation for the expected 2014
spike in primary-care demand. The commission was supposed
to explore workforce needs in rural and medically under-served
settings, behavioral health, the nursing workforce capacity,
graduate medical education (GME) policies, and education and
loan programs for health-care professionals.

The panel has never met, and is unlikely to because it remains
unfunded because of Republican opposition to Obamacare. Its
15 members were appointed in September 2010 by the U.S.
comptroller general. Ten of the members' terms subsequently expired, and they were reappointed for another three years
each—although it is not clear toward what end.

Direct effects of ACA expansion

The Affordable Care Act's (ACA) 2014 increase in newly

CURRENT SITUATION

Q: Which of the following best describes your current practice?

I am at full capacity
·· 52.7%

I have time to see more patients and assume more duties
······················ 24.6%

I am overextended and overworked
······················ 22.7%

Source: : Physicians Foundation Survey of America's Physicians, 2012.

About 3 out of 4 physician practices are at or over capacity.

insured patients is arriving at a time when the U.S. already has a shortage of more than 15,000 primary-care physicians and hospital emergency visits are rising at twice the rate of population growth. The Congressional Budget Office estimated that up to 22 million previously uninsured non elderly Americans would gain health insurance by 2014, and that number may reach 26 million or more by 2022. Many of the newly insured will be arriving with long-unmet needs for care.

Of those, more than one-third did not seek care in the year prior of being surveyed and nearly half lacked a regular healthcare provider.

Policy researchers have estimated that the insurance added under the ACA will produce 15 million to 24 million additional primary-care visits annually.

Meanwhile, physicians are slowly backing away. Their

average workweek decreased from 55 hours in 1996 to 51 hours in 2008. That is the equivalent of losing 36,000 additional doctors in a decade. The financial incentive to work harder, they say, is simply no longer there.

Only one out of four physicians say they will work as hard in three years as they do now. The remainder say they will cut back their hours, retire or seek nonclinical employment. The recession prompted many to delay retirement. The health-care industry experienced the largest decline in retirement rates of all economic sectors. In 2009-10, about 1.5 percent of full-time health-care workers retired compared with 4 percent in 2004-07. The retirement rate inevitably will increase. One out of four U.S. physicians is age 60 or older.

Most experts point to the ACA for the worsening primary-care physician shortage. However, *Annals of Family Medicine* researchers took a contrarian view: Population growth and aging, more than insurance expansion, will drive shortages. They estimate the U.S. will need nearly 52,000 more primary-care physicians by 2025. They attributed more than 33,000 of that number to population growth, 10,000 to aging and 8,000 to the ACA's insurance expansion.

The number of those over age 65 is expected to grow by about 45 percent from 2013 through 2025, compared with about a 6 percent for the U.S. during that period. Between 2010 and 2030, 27 million more Americans are expected to have hypertension, 8 million more with coronary heart disease and 3 million with heart failure. The elderly population with Alzheimer's disease is expected to increase 40 percent by 2025, and a 21 percent increase is expected for elderly people with diagnosed diabetes.

Even safety-net physicians will be hard pressed to care for

CUTTING BACK

Q: In the next one to three years, do you plan to _____?

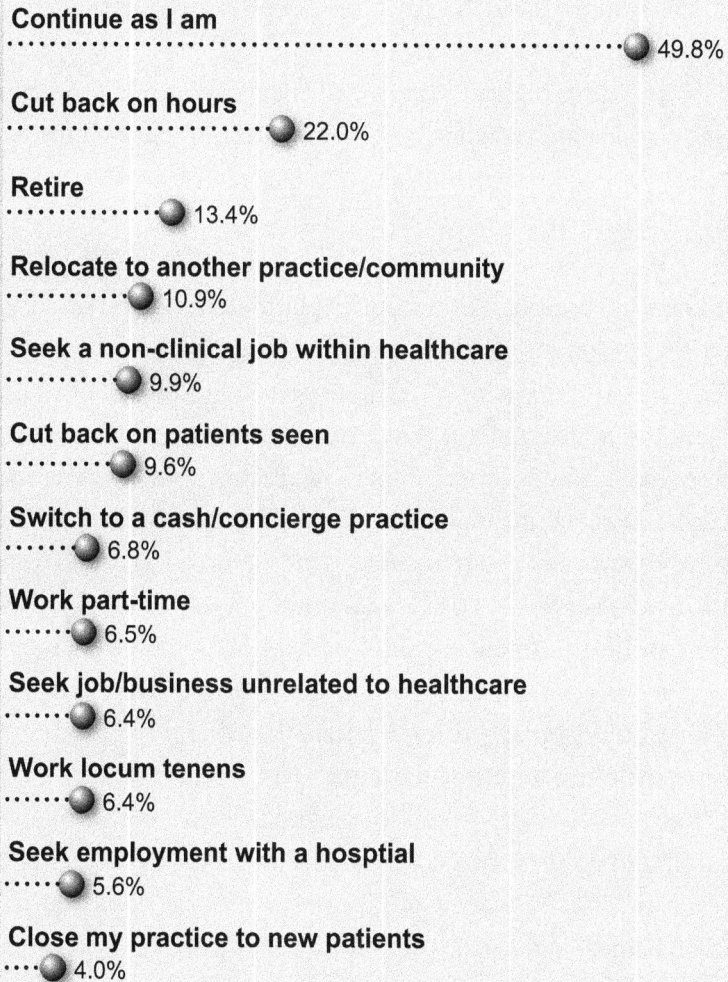

Continue as I am
··· 49.8%

Cut back on hours
···················· 22.0%

Retire
············· 13.4%

Relocate to another practice/community
············ 10.9%

Seek a non-clinical job within healthcare
············ 9.9%

Cut back on patients seen
··········· 9.6%

Switch to a cash/concierge practice
········ 6.8%

Work part-time
········ 6.5%

Seek job/business unrelated to healthcare
········ 6.4%

Work locum tenens
········ 6.4%

Seek employment with a hosptial
······· 5.6%

Close my practice to new patients
····· 4.0%

Source: Physicians Foundation Survey of America's Physicians, 2012.

Half of the nation's physicians plan to reduce their workloads over the next three years.

newly insured patients in 2014. A study by researchers at the Mongan Institute for Health Policy at Massachusetts General Hospital found that a significant percentage of the primary-care physicians most likely to care for newly insured patients may not accept new patients.

About half of Massachusetts internists and family physicians are not accepting new patients. Wait times for new patients to get an appointment with a family physician increased from 29 days in 2010 to 45 days in 2012.

The onslaught of newly insured will not be nearly as great as first feared. About half of the states planned not to expand their Medicaid programs in 2014. If so, it means that 5.3 million fewer low-income people would gain access to this public insurance option. As an alternative, about two out of three of those would qualify for subsidies on the ACA's health-insurance exchanges.

Regardless, nearly half of U.S. physicians say they will be unable to take on newly insured patients under the ACA, according to a survey by CareCloud and QuantiaMD.

The millions of newly insured may allow some physicians to be pickier about their clientele. More than one out of four physicians would stop accepting insurers that do not pay well even if it meant firing longtime patients.

About four out of 10 said they would not drop a low-paying insurer, and 32 percent said "it depends." Survey comments indicated that those who would drop an insurer would do so if reimbursement did not cover practice expenses. Those who said they would keep a low-paying insurer said they felt an obligation to treat all patients.

The question is whether the influx of newly insured will lower the acceptance rate for lower-paying government insurance or result in overworked staff. A significant portion of the physician workforce already is overextended.

According to a *JAMA Internal Medicine* study, hospital physicians said they safely could attend to 15 patients per shift. However, nearly half said their typical workload exceeded that level.

The ACA could further strain hospital workloads as they simultaneously cut costs and manage the influx of new patients. "Society needs to reduce health-care costs, but do so wisely," the study's authors wrote. "Hospitals need to create standards for safe levels of work.... Excessively increasing the workload may lead to suboptimal care and less direct patient-care time, which may paradoxically increase, rather than decrease, costs."

Todd Atwater, chief executive officer of the South Carolina Medical Association, said the newly insured will be more of an issue for hospitals because Medicaid is not being expanded in his state to ease the burden of uncompensated care.

In 2012, more than 8 out of 10 office-based physicians were accepting Medicare patients, while two-thirds accepted Medicaid patients. About 69 percent of primary-care physicians accepted Medicare, compared with about 83 percent of specialists.

The acceptance of government insurance became more common as the number of physicians in a practice increased. Nearly nine out of 10 hospital-owned practices accepted Medicare and Medicaid.

The Government Accountability Office (GAO) reported in late 2012 that Medicaid offices were having trouble finding enough providers to care for Medicaid patients. The shortage is most acute among dentists. Specialists came in second, followed by mental-health and substance-abuse providers and primary-care physicians.

The GAO conducted the impact of Medicaid enrollment's significant growth in recent years because of the economic downturn—growth that is only expected to accelerate because of the ACA's 2014 Medicaid expansion.

The GAO and the Washington-based Center for Studying Health System Change contend, nevertheless, that the expansion of Medicaid coverage will not overwhelm the nation's physicians.

They cited the fact that the creation of the Children's Health Insurance Program (CHIP) in 1997 did not create a deluge of patients overwhelming the nation's pediatricians. The researchers found that pediatricians actually reduced their work hours. In fact, they found that a 5 percent increase in the share of children enrolled in CHIP was associated with a 14 percent decline in pediatrician work hours. They speculated that CHIP cut average reimbursement rates for pediatricians that led them to reduce their hours, or shorter hours reflected the managed-care gatekeeper nature of CHIP.

Skeptics point out that the CHIP expansion was nowhere near that of the ACA in scope and there likely had been little pent-up health-care demand by the newly insured children.

Diagnostic errors and time pressure

Diagnostic errors are plentiful in primary care, because there are a half-billion often-hasty visits a year—leaving lots of opportunity for misdiagnosis.

Research on diagnostic mistakes suggests that most primary-care misdiagnoses are related to basic elements of the office visit. Time constraints make it harder for physicians to solve the medical mysteries that confront them.

Missed, incorrect or delayed diagnoses were most frequent in conditions common in primary-care settings, including pneumonia, congestive heart failure, acute renal failure, cancer and urinary tract infections, according to one study.

The study's authors said diagnostic errors are likely to remain a nettlesome problem as long as providers are pressured to keep visits short and make decisions quickly—a growing threat with 2014's insurance expansion. Breakdowns during the clinician-patient encounter—including an inadequate record of a patient's medical history and failure to review previous documentation—were to blame for more than three out of four errors. The risk of "moderate" to "severe" harm was evident in nearly all of the misdiagnoses.

Errors in diagnosis are responsible for more deaths, disabilities and medical liability payments than any other kind of medical error.

Johns Hopkins researchers found that diagnostic errors—not surgical mistakes or medication overdoses—accounted for the largest fraction of claims, the most severe patient harm and the highest total of penalty payouts. Diagnosis-related payments amounted to $38.8 billion between 1986 and 2010, according to a review of more than 100,000 medical liability cases. Errors in diagnosis, nearly 30 percent of the total, compares with 27 percent for treatment mistakes and 24 percent for surgical errors.

Researchers estimated that misdiagnosis kills or permanently injures 80,000 to 160,000 Americans annually.

"This is more evidence that diagnostic errors could easily be the biggest patient safety and medical malpractice problem in the United States," said Dr. David E. Newman-Toker, M.D., an associate professor of neurology at the Johns Hopkins University School of Medicine and leader of the study.

A 2003 JAMA study found that about 5 percent of U.S. autopsies uncovered diagnoses that, if made when the patient was alive, could have saved the patient's life.

The likely glut of patients beginning in 2014 will have patients spilling into other sites of care. Retailers are gearing up to accept them with open arms. Walgreens announced in April 2013 that it would become the first retail chain to expand its health-care services to include diagnosis and treatment of patients for chronic conditions such as diabetes, high cholesterol and asthma. The company said it planned to use nurse practitioners (NPs) and physician assistants (PAs) in 300 clinics in 18 states and the District of Columbia.

Consumers are attracted by the retail clinics' convenience, transparent pricing and cost savings. Costs are about 30 to 40 percent lower than in physician offices and 80 percent cheaper than at a hospital emergency department. According to a 2013 Harris Poll, more than one out of four U.S. adults said they used a walk-in retail clinic or work-based clinic in the past two years—more than triple the rate in 2008.

Ongoing fight over scope of practice

NPs often are suggested as a relief valve for the primary-care physician shortage. Their ranks are growing much faster. Between 1990 and 2012, the physician workforce grew 50 percent while that of NPS and PAs increased fivefold. NPs' average salaries are less than half those of physicians', and they provide comparable quality, according to several research studies.

However, adding an NP can be less cost-effective than

IN THE NEXT ONE TO THREE YEARS, DO YOU PLAN TO . . .

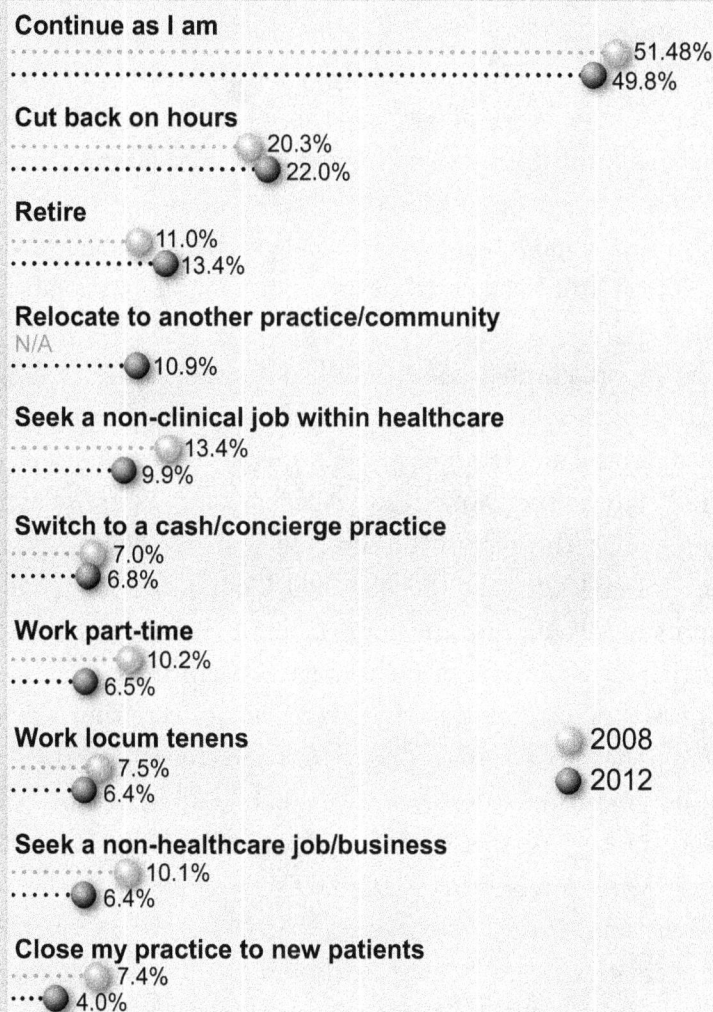

Continue as I am
51.48%
49.8%

Cut back on hours
20.3%
22.0%

Retire
11.0%
13.4%

Relocate to another practice/community
N/A
10.9%

Seek a non-clinical job within healthcare
13.4%
9.9%

Switch to a cash/concierge practice
7.0%
6.8%

Work part-time
10.2%
6.5%

Work locum tenens
7.5%
6.4%

2008
2012

Seek a non-healthcare job/business
10.1%
6.4%

Close my practice to new patients
7.4%
4.0%

Source: Physicians Foundation Survey of America's Physicians, 2012.

In the next one to three years, more than half of physicians plan to cut back on patients, work part-time, switch to concierge medicine, retire or take other steps that would reduce patient access to their services adding a physician, because of scope-of-practice limits. NPs may increase care volume, but cases that are more complex require a second visit with a physician. That physician oversight takes away from a practice's capacity to see more patients.

NPs can practice independently of a physician in 16 states.

The American Academy of Family Physicians (AAFP) lashed out at the notion that NPs and PAs could fill the gap created by the growing physician shortage. AAFP released a report in 2012 saying more nurse-led medical practices were not a viable solution. It instead urged the creation of more physician-led PCMHs.

The report pointed out that NPs had an average of 5,350 hours of training, compared with 21,700 hours for physicians in medical school and residency.

Predictably, the American Academy of Nurse Practitioners called the report "misdirected and out of step." The group pointed out that the National Committee for Quality Assurance, URAC and the Joint Commission do not require physician leadership for medical-home recognition.

There is no dispute that there is a primary-care shortage, at least in under-served areas. There is less agreement over the role of other practitioners—specifically PAs and advanced-practice nurses—in keeping the ACA from breaking the back of an already strained primary-care system.

American Medical Association (AMA) analysts say they have seen an increase in state legislation to allow broader scope of practice since the ACA was passed. Nearly 1,800 bills related to scope of practice were introduced in states in 2011-12. Nearly 150 were introduced in just the first few weeks of 2013, according to the National Conference of State Legislatures.

More than four out of five NPs say they should be able to lead medical homes and receive the same pay as physicians for providing the same clinical services. Only one out of five physicians agreed with NPs on either issue. Only one out of four NPs believed physicians delivered a "higher quality of examination and consultation," compared with two out of three physicians who agreed with the statement.

A 2010 Institute of Medicine report urged expansion of scope of practice for advanced-practice nurses to counteract primary-care shortages.

A systematic review of 26 studies published since 2000 found that health status of patients, treatment practices and prescribing behavior were consistent between physicians and NPs. Patients who saw NPs also were more satisfied with their care.

In a provocative *Health Affairs* study, researchers said the physician shortage was overestimated and could be avoided by the proper deployment of physicians and mid-level clinicians.

A RAND Corp. study asserted that much of the primary-care shortage could be eliminated if the nation increased its use of new models of care that expanded the roles of NPs and PAs. Researchers said expansion of PCMHs and nurse-managed health centers could help eliminate half of the shortage by 2025. If medical homes delivered 50 percent of primary care—compared with the current 15 percent—the shortage would fall by 25 percent. If nurse-managed health centers expanded to account for 5 percent of primary care—compared with 0.5 percent now—the shortage would fall by another 25 percent, the researchers said. Expansion of patient-centered medical homes and nurse-managed health centers could help eliminate 50 percent or more of the primary-care physician shortage expected to face the U.S.

by 2025, they said.

Researchers at Columbia Business School in New York and the University of Pennsylvania's Wharton School say the traditional ratio of one physician for every 2,500 patients is an outmoded metric.

They said team care that included "pooled" physicians, NPs, PAs and technology that could reduce physician office visits would enable larger patient panels, and doing so would make the impending physician shortage "virtually evaporate."

Regardless of the division over scope of practice, medical groups and health-care organizations do not deny the value of non-physician practitioners. They plan to increase their recruitment of them and compensate them more generously, according to an American Medical Group Association survey of health systems, hospitals and practices. More than half increased their recruitment of mid-level clinicians in 2012 and planned to do so again in 2013, and two out of three increased their compensation in the past 12 months.

Primary-care shortages will worsen

The U.S. has about the same number of physicians per capita as other industrialized nations. However, the U.S. has far fewer primary-care physicians. They make up about 50 percent of the physician workforce in most other developed nations, compared with 35 percent in the U.S.

This is reflected in the time it takes to see a doctor. A study of 11 industrialized nations found that 80 percent of Americans could get in to see a specialist within four weeks. Only Germany had a better rate. However, only 57 percent of Americans could see a primary-care doctor the same day or the next day.

That compares with 93 percent in Switzerland and 70 percent in Great Britain, whose system is often erroneously branded as "socialized medicine." The shorter supply of primary-care doctors—the ones you need in a hurry—means slower service in the U.S. The number of U.S. specialists per capita has risen dramatically since 1965, while the ratio of primary-care physicians to the general population has remained relatively constant. The outlook is for more of the same: greater scarcity of primary care and a growing supply of specialists.

The primary-care workload is expected to increase by nearly 30 percent between 2005 and 2025. A number of factors feed this demand, including a population growth of about 20 percent, a flood of baby boomers becoming Medicare beneficiaries and acquiring medical conditions as they age, and 30 million more Americans with Medicaid or subsidized insurance.

However, the supply of primary-care physicians is expected to rise by only 2 to 7 percent. Three out of four primary-care physicians say they already are at or over capacity. The math screams that there will be a crisis of health-care access in the next 15 years. Expect longer waits for appointments, shorter physician visits, greater use of non physicians for routine care, and higher prices. The U.S. trains about 16,000 doctors a year. The nation would have to increase that number by 6,000 to 8,000 annually for 20 years to meet expected demand.

Some still believe there is an oversupply of physicians, leading to over treatment and expression of Parkinson's Law: "Work expands to fill the time available for its completion."

In any case, primary-care physician jobs have become more difficult to fill.

According to the Association of Staff Physician Recruiters,

primary-care physician positions took 151 days to fill in 2011, up from 125 in 2010 and 115 in 2009.

One of the effects of the shortage is that new primary-care physicians earned a starting median salary of $180,000 in 2012, compared with $175,000 the previous year.

Over a lifetime, a primary-care physician can expect to make $1.5 million less than a medical school classmate who becomes a specialist. The gap can rise as high as $2.8 million if that classmate becomes a neurosurgeon.

As Princeton economist Uwe Reinhardt wrote in a *New York Times* blog, "Surely there is something absurd when a nation pays a primary-care physician poorly relative to other specialists and then wrings its hands over a shortage of primary-care physicians."

Fewer than half of primary-care physicians are paid for hospital call coverage. In contrast, about 80 percent of surgical specialists are paid to be on call.

Young doctors simply are not choosing general medicine careers. Only one out of 14 of today's medical students want to be a primary-care physician, according to one study. About 3,600 graduating residents are choosing a general internist career, compared with more than 10,700 who are choosing a sub specialty. Of those choosing a generalist career path as first-year residents, only slightly more than half will stay on that path through their third year of residency.

Lead author Colin West said there were two main factors in why so few internal-medicine residents were planning a primary-care career: They were taking training wherever they could get it, and they see something negative about primary care or something attractive about a subspecialty career.

He said his findings suggest that increasing the number of medical colleges and primary-care residency slots will simply produce more subspecialists unless primary care is made more attractive. And if the number of sub-specialist GME slots were limited, there would be more physicians in primary care who would rather be doing something else.

More than half of the nation's physicians are over 50 years old, according to the Federation of State Medical Boards.

Government efforts to avert the worsening shortage of primary-care physicians have largely failed.

In 2003, the Medicare Prescription Drug, Improvement and Modernization Act attempted to redistribute about 3,000 residency positions in U.S. hospitals to primary-care positions and to rural areas.

However, of more than 300 hospitals that received additional residency positions, only 12 appointments were in rural areas. Meanwhile, the relative growth of specialist training doubled.

The U.S. government provides hospitals with almost $13 billion annually to help support medical residencies. Medicare paid $9.7 billion for GME training in 2009. Medicaid chipped in almost $4 billion a year, and the U.S. Department of Veterans Affairs contributed $800 million annually.

Together, the cost of funding graduate medical education represents the largest public investment in health-care workforce development.

Only 2 percent of medical students in a 2011 study said they planned to practice primary care as a general internist. Over the past two decades, medical students have acquired more debt and are more aware of internal medicine's higher workload and stress, as well as lower pay.

Many are expecting patients who cannot get physician appointments to go to emergency departments (ED). However, that has been happening for several years.

Hospital admissions from the ED increased by 17 percent over seven years, in part because primary-care physicians often rely on the emergency physicians to evaluate and hospitalize their most complex and sickest patients. Four out of five who contacted their primary-care physician or other medical provider before seeking emergency care were told to go directly to the ED.

For this and other reasons, primary-care physicians generate more revenue for their affiliated hospitals than specialists do —$1.57 million per year vs. $1.42 million, respectively.

Relying on international physicians

The U.S. increasingly outsourced its primary care because of poor income prospects. Primary-care physicians' income essentially has stayed the same since the 1990s, while their practice expenses have steadily increased. After accounting for inflation, their average income fell 7 percent from 1995 to 2003. This obviously is an unsustainable business model.

Primary-care physicians' share of the U.S. health-care dollar is only seven cents. Even if payers cut reimbursement for physician services by 25 percent—certainly a doomsday scenario for doctors—the average rate of medical inflation would decrease from 6.2 percent to 5.7 percent.

However, primary-care doctors control 80 cents of the health-care dollar by sending their patients to hospitals, referring them to specialists and handing out prescriptions. This is a key paradox: Primary-care physicians arguably are the most powerful players in the health-care system but are under appreciated and comparatively undercompensated. In a 2006 survey, nearly eight out of 10 characterized themselves as "junior partners" or "second-class citizens" in the health-care galaxy. Medical students, including those who plan to become primary-care physicians, view the work more negatively than that of other physicians.

First-year guaranteed compensation for specialty physicians is $240,000 to $260,000, compared with about $180,000 for primary-care physicians. There is a perception that surgeons endure greater mental challenges and stress than primary-care physicians, which some believe accounts for the income disparity. However, a group of University of Cincinnati scientists used work-intensity measurement tools to determine that the mental burden was similar.

About one out of four physicians practicing in the U.S. and 10 to 15 percent of those in residency programs are international medical graduates (IMGs).

The nation's medical schools are on track to increase enrollment by 30 percent in 2016 compared with 2005, a goal called for by the Association of American Medical Colleges (AAMC). However, association president Darrell Kirch noted, "This won't amount to a single new doctor in practice without an expansion of residency positions."

In 2013, the number of first-year medical students exceeded 20,000 for the first time.

Despite the fact that most physicians said they would not recommend the profession to their children, applicants flooded medical school admissions offices in record numbers in 2012, according to the AAMC. The applicant pool has grown nearly every year for the past decade.

However, the number of residency positions has not expanded

and, in fact, may contract because of decreases in GME funding.

IMGs play a significant role in treating vulnerable populations. They have an oversized presence in counties with high infant mortality and lower socioeconomic status, and in those designated as rural. They tend to work more in the public sector and labor for longer hours. They are twice as likely to work in medically under-served areas as U.S. medical graduates are. They account for more than one out of three physicians in shortage areas, and one out of 10 U.S. hospitals are highly dependent on them.

The AMA House of Delegates urged the expansion of the J-1 visa waiver program. It allocates 30 positions for international medical school graduates who complete graduate medical education and agree to work in federally designated shortage areas in exchange for waivers from the return-home visa requirement.

The delegates also urged the AMA to lobby to protect pediatric GME slots, for which funding must be approved by Congress. The program was targeted for $48.5 million in cuts in the Obama administration's budget for fiscal year 2011, although that was avoided. Children's hospitals train 40 percent of pediatricians and 43 percent of pediatric specialists.

No more docs without more GME slots

The battle is on to defend and expand the nation's GME slots. Teaching hospitals quadrupled their lobbying budget in 2011, to $2.8 million, according to the Center for Responsive Politics. They are pushing legislation that would add 3,000 residencies annually through 2017. The price tag: $9 billion.

Nearly half of medical school deans expressed "major concern" about nationwide enrollment growing faster than graduate medical education, and 33 percent reported it as a "major concern" in their state.

The other problem: Those in the pipeline will not help in dealing with the 2014 wave of new patients.

With at least 12 new schools opening and existing ones growing, enrollment is expected to create 5,000 more graduates a year by 2019.

Medicare-funded GME spots essentially have remained frozen since the Balanced Budget Act of 1997.

There currently are more residency openings than U.S. allopathic medical school graduates. The gap traditionally has been filled by graduates of U.S. osteopathic schools and foreign medical schools.

At the current expansion rate, graduates from U.S. medical and osteopathic schools alone will exceed the number of expected residencies by the end of the decade, according to AAMC. The U.S. is expected to graduate more than 27,000 medical students in 2020, which is 50 percent more than in 2000. If residency programs had not been capped in 1997 and GME slots had been allowed to grow at their historical rate, there would be no physician shortage today.

Residency applicants from foreign schools are likely to be squeezed out. Graduates of foreign medical schools now make up more than 25 percent of the U.S. physician workforce—and about half of primary-care doctors—because U.S. graduates gravitate toward specialties that are more lucrative. Foreign doctors also make up a disproportionate share of those in rural communities and public clinics, and they treat a higher share of minority patients.

Despite this, there have been multiple proposals to slash GME funding because of ongoing federal budget deficit-reduction efforts. GME reductions as high as 50 percent have been recommended by the Medicare Payment Advisory Commission and the National Commission on Fiscal Responsibility and Reform, as well as President Obama's 2013 budget proposal.

The AAMC estimated in 2011 that a 50 percent reduction in Medicare GME funding would result in the closing of 2,551 residency and fellowship programs and the loss of 33,023 GME positions.

About nine out of 10 allopathic and osteopathic medicine graduates had educational debt in 2011. The average debt is $205,674 for osteopathic students and $162,000 for allopathic students.

A medical school graduate with $162,000 of debt would have monthly payments ranging from $1,500 to $2,100 after residency training, depending on the repayment plan, according to the AAMC.

Vanishing Autonomy

R ipley Hollister has been president of his county's medical society in Colorado Springs and a director of the Colorado Medical Society. He has been a unit commander of the Medical Reserve Corps of El Paso County. His practice has a world-class view of the Rocky Mountains from its floor-to-ceiling windows.

Hollister also does the laundry for his medical practice each weeknight. "Is that the way it should be?" he asks.

Being a launderer has nothing to do with providing high-quality patient care. It has everything to do with economic survival. It is also emblematic of the menial nonclinical tasks, so common now, that erode physician autonomy.

Hollister has practiced cradle-to-grave primary care his entire career. He literally built a practice in a two-acre cornfield in Ramer, Tenn., to satisfy his National Health Service Corps commitment and wipe out what would have been a $300,000 medical-school debt. The town, population 354, is in McNairy County, where Sheriff Buford Pusser, the subject of the *Walking Tall* movie series, fought moonshining, prostitution and gambling near the Mississippi state line in the late 1960s.

Hollister has had his solo practice for 16 years. Two mid-level providers help him care for 4,700 patients. He has trimmed his workweek to about 50 hours and no longer does obstetrics.

Hollister said falling reimbursement rates and rising practice expenses inevitably mean he must shrink his practice. Marginal clinical services cease. He stopped doing colonoscopies because revenue from them barely covered his expenses. When equipment broke down or needed to be upgraded, he simply stopped providing the service because he could not justify the expense. Lab tests, once done on site, are now outsourced. Results are slow to return. Patients are inconvenienced.

Hollister has stopped doing immunizations. "I discovered I lost $40 on every vaccination. I can't do that. People can't understand why they can't get vaccinated at the doctor's office. I send them to Wal-Mart or Walgreens. They buy in volume. I can't. So I send them elsewhere. "

Hollister is well aware that he is part of a vanishing breed of physician: the solo practitioner who is working hard to serve a larger purpose.

Doctors "are tight-lipped," he said. "They won't tell you they are going under. They just vanish. They get taken over by a larger entity: hospitals, health plans, government. You see a wave of doctors who see this as a safe harbor. But hospitals are still finding they can't manage doctors and make money. So they cut back doctors' salaries or tell them to see more patients.

"The older ones are being pushed out (of the system). Many are pissed off and leaving. They have a different view of medicine than the new ones. Being a doctor defined who they were. It was their purpose in life. Younger doctors work maybe 40 hours a

PHYSICIAN INFLUENCE ON HEALTH SYSTEM

Q: Physicians have little influence on the direction of healthcare and have little ability to effect change. Do you . . .?

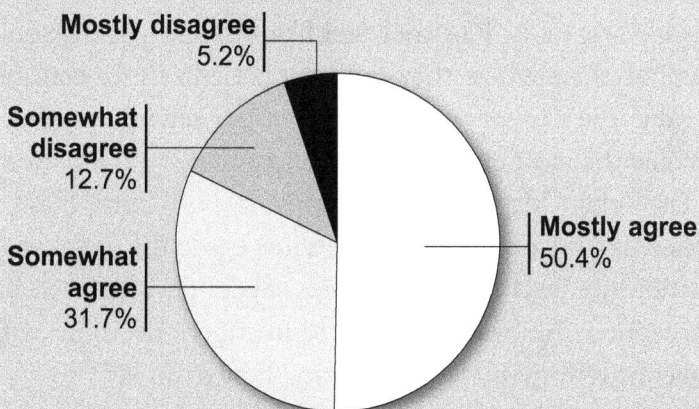

Mostly disagree
5.2%

Somewhat
disagree
12.7%

Somewhat
agree
31.7%

Mostly agree
50.4%

Source: Physicians Foundation Survey of America's Physicians, 2012.

More than 8 out of 10 physicians believe doctors have little ability to change the health-care system.

week. They see it more as employment than a profession. They have a different view about quality of life. They won't be quite the workforce (in quantity of hours)," he said.

Despite his profession's head winds, Hollister has no plans to retire. "I want to be practicing as long as I am mentally crisp. I'm never retiring, but I could be forced (by administrative or practice burdens). I just need a support staff and a place to work."

Autonomy diminishing

Physicians who say they are dissatisfied with their jobs list decreasing autonomy as the No. 1 reason.

Nearly half cited that, compared with one out of three who named low reimbursement and one out of four who blamed administrative hassles, according to a Jackson Healthcare survey.

"Physicians are working harder and longer hours for less reimbursement," Richard Jackson, chairman and CEO of Jackson Healthcare, said. "Plus they feel like insurers, government and hospitals dictate how they can treat patients. If we continue to devalue the experience and skills of our physicians, they will become the most expensive data entry clerks in the nation. "

Dr. Robert Monteiro, an internist in New Bern, N.C., said, "There is a huge amount of interference into the doctor-patient relationship, and that has a large impact on your professional satisfaction. You want to come to treatment decisions without someone telling you what to do and how to do it."

Monteiro said preauthorization for medications, imaging and treatments requires increasing amounts of time. He said the uncompensated time required to complete paperwork associated with patient care limits patient access, because physicians run out of hours. He added that the constantly shifting insurance-plan changes and requirements can be overwhelming.

"It's as if you are playing a game and don't know the rules. Then rules constantly change and maybe you get penalized for new rules, even if you don't know what they are. As doctors, we have no problem justifying how we take care of patients. But having to fill out a three-page form to get a generic blood thinner is ridiculous," he said.

Don Alexander, former chief executive officer of the Tennessee Medical Association, said, "Doctors go into medicine to treat patients with the best knowledge they have and best tools they have at their disposal. When they lose the ability to treat or diagnose patients like they've been trained to do, they lose that autonomy. The wedge between doctor and patient gets bigger. When you hinder a doctor's independent judgment, you're hindering the best medical care that's out there."

Dr. Joseph Valenti, an obstetrician and gynecologist in Denton, Texas, said he has had the same contract with Blue Cross Blue Shield of Texas for five years. He said he tried to create a new contract with quality incentives. The company turned down his request, he said, despite the fact that the insurer considered his quality of care excellent.

"They said, 'Since you're doing everything right, you don't need more money.' This is the worst sort of antithetical thinking. Why am I trying so hard? I should just do a crappy job so I can get more money from them (by subsequently improving quality). Doctors have no power. The insurance companies and hospitals have all the power," he said.

Robert Seligson, chief executive officer of the North Carolina Medical Society, said lack of autonomy is the biggest barrier physicians face.

"Doctors did not get in on the major system reforms. They were put in the back of the bus. The ACA was done with insufficient doctor input. It was drafted by people who either have not been in the real world or don't have to worry about where the next paycheck is coming from. I feel doctors should have been leading the charge," he said.

A clash of goals

In a *Journal of the American Medical Association* (JAMA) analysis, Hamilton Moses III argued that forces within the U.S. health-care system create a triangle of tension among patient desire for choice, personal attention and unbiased guidance; physician goals of professionalism and autonomy; and public and private payer objectives of aggregate economic value across large populations. He asserted that physician autonomy is in conflict with hospital and insurance consolidation, and population health—which he called "Big Med," "Big Pay," and "Big Data."

"Measurements of cost and outcome (applied to groups) are supplanting individuals' preferences. Clinicians increasingly are expected to substitute social and economic goals for the needs of a single patient," Moses wrote.

The American Medical Association (AMA) commissioned the RAND Corp. to get a better handle on why physician morale is declining. Researchers conducted hundreds of interviews across six states. They found that physicians' perceptions of their ability to deliver high-quality care determined their satisfaction levels. Physicians expressed exasperation with multiple barriers to delivering that care: administrative hassles, the pressure to see more patients to meet rising practice expenses, and frustrating electronic health record systems. All of these factors were nibbling at their ability and freedom to give patients what they considered the best possible care.

Physicians facing decisions about their practices have to consider the inevitable loss of clinical autonomy that comes with joining health systems and large practices that can negotiate more favorable third-party payer contracts.

Steve Corso, Texas-based MedSynergies' managing director of physician engagement, has seen the effects of lost autonomy as health systems try to absorb newly acquired physicians.

He said, "Older agreements included physician autonomy.

PHYSICIAN INCOME

Q: Describe your income from the practice of medicine over the last three years.

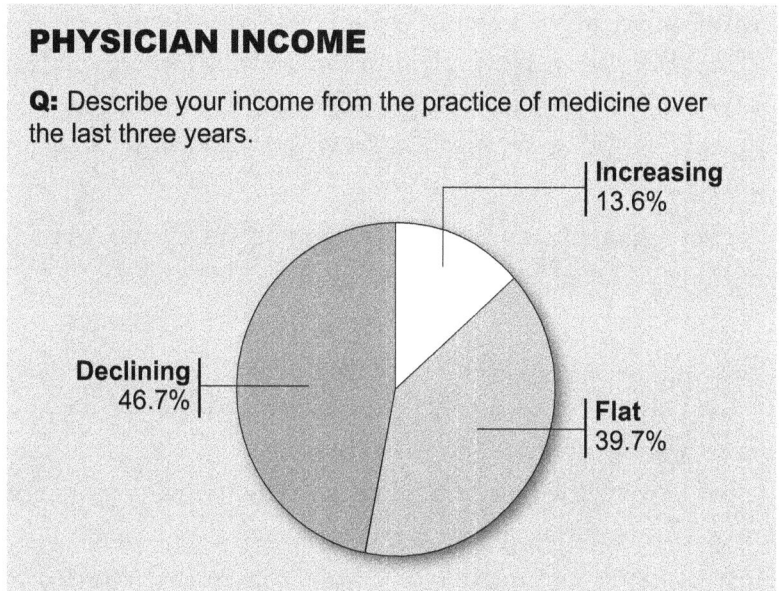

Increasing 13.6%

Declining 46.7%

Flat 39.7%

Source: Physicians Foundation Survey of America's Physicians, 2012.

Physician income has been flat or declining in the last three years for nearly 9 out of 10 U.S. physicians.

The reality now is that physician acquisition means centralization, and that's not autonomy. Losing autonomy is the root cause of anxiety for physicians."

Gary Price, a plastic surgeon in Guilford, Conn., said, "There is no question that my ability to directly control my patients in a hospital environment has been eroded. This has been going on for 10 years. The size of the health systems and state and federal regulatory burden make it more difficult for doctors to effect change in that environment. The regulatory issues lead to people who are not physicians supervising physicians who have no choice otherwise."

Todd Atwater, chief executive officer of the South Carolina Medical Association, said physician autonomy takes a hit when doctors move into a hospital setting.

"An ACO is an HMO, with a hospital on top rather than an insurer. As payment becomes capitated, you may see doctor behavior change and more affected by decisions of the system," he said.

Physicians are being left out of hospital efforts to improve the patient experience, according to a Beryl Institute survey.

Only 3 percent of health-care executives said physicians or other clinicians held primary responsibility and accountability for the patient experience. Only 1 percent said chief medical officers were in charge.

The idea of "the patient experience," composed of strategies designed to improve patient satisfaction and outcomes, continues to gain more traction as payment increasingly is tied to quality. Improving the patient experience is emerging as a top priority among U.S. hospital systems.

The patient experience encompasses care coordination, provider communication with caregivers and staff responsiveness. More than one out of four executives surveyed said they believed physicians did not support—and were a major roadblock to—improving the patient experience.

In November 2012, the AMA House of Delegates established six principles to guide newly employed physicians and their employers.

The principles addressed potentially problematic aspects of the employer-employee relationship, including conflicts of interest, advocacy, contracting, hospital-medical staff relations, peer review and performance evaluations, and payment agreements.

Dr. Joseph P. Annis, an AMA board member, said, "The

guidelines reinforce that patients' welfare must take priority in any situation where the interests of physicians and employers conflict."

Among other points in the policy statement:

- Although a physician's paramount responsibility is to patients, he or she owes loyalty to the employer, and this "divided loyalty" could lead to conflicts of interest, such as financial incentives to over treat or under treat patients.
- Physicians should always make treatment and referral decisions based on the best interests of the patients. Patients should be told whenever a hospital provides financial incentives that encourage, discourage or restrict referrals or treatment options.

Dr. Jerry Kennett, a leader of the American College of Cardiology, told *The New York Times* that he had been told doctors were instructed not to place defibrillators in Medicaid patients because "it's a money-losing proposition" for the hospital. He also said physicians were told they had to use the hospital's imaging and lab facilities despite the fact that they could get better quality elsewhere.

Dissatisfaction over pay

Physician pay accounts for less than 9 percent of U.S. health-care costs, the second-lowest percentage among physicians in nine Western nations.

Primary-care physicians are the least satisfied of those in all major specialties. Fewer than half said they would again select primary care if they were choosing a specialty today. Orthopedic surgeons, radiologists, anesthesiologists and cardiologists make, on average, twice the income of primary-care physicians.

Few physicians consider themselves rich, and only about half believe they are fairly compensated.

Four of 10 physicians said their take-home pay declined from 2011 to 2012, and more than half believe their incomes will fall substantially in the next one to three years. Nearly 20 percent of physicians said their income fell more than 10 percent. Of those who said their income dropped, nearly 40 percent blamed the Affordable Care Act (ACA).

The 2012 Physicians Foundation survey found similar results. More than 86 percent of physicians said income in their practices has been flat or declining in the previous three years.

Physician salary growth trailed that of other health-care professionals between 1987 and 2010. Physician incomes grew 24 percent between 1982 and 1989, and decreased 7.1 percent between 1995 and 2003.

Between 2006 and 2010, professionals in other health-care fields—including dentists, nurses and pharmacists—saw a 44 percent average salary increase, compared with a 9.6 percent increase in physicians' salaries.

Physicians were expected to get an average 2.4 percent raise in 2014, with hospital-employed physicians receiving an even lower raise, according to a physician compensation survey.

Reimbursement cuts have been deep in cardiology. For example, Medicare cut payments for nuclear scans by about 40 percent in 2010.

The cuts have changed the employment landscape dramatically for cardiology practices. In Wisconsin, the share of heart doctors who are in private practice fell to 11 percent, compared with 62 percent in 2007. According to consultant MedAxiom, nearly eight out of 10 U.S. cardiology groups were either integrated into hospitals, in the process of being integrated or considering it.

About one out of three surgeons were self-employed in 2009, compared with about half in 2001. Full-time employment in hospitals was up by about one-third, with the trend especially pronounced among younger surgeons and female surgeons.

Physicians often are criticized for their lofty incomes. However, patients apparently believe that their own doctors are underpaid. For example, hip-replacement patients thought their physician should be paid $14,358 for the procedure and guessed that Medicare paid $8,212. The actual amount was $1,375. Orthopedic surgeons specializing in joint surgery earn slightly more than $600,000 a year. If they earned what their patients thought they should, annual salaries would be about $63 million.

Women physicians make less than men. Two Yale researchers calculated that for more than half of female doctors, the net present value of becoming a primary-care physician was less than that of becoming a physician assistant. That is indicative of the relatively low income of female primary-care physicians, as well as the burdensome medical-school debts they acquire.

All physicians are feeling constrained by rising practice costs and reimbursement trends. According to a 2013 MGMA survey, the No. 1 challenge of running a physician practice was dealing with rising operating costs, followed by the uncertainty of possible Medicare reimbursement cuts, new models of health-care delivery and the increasing difficulty of collecting from patients with high-deductible health plans.

Unwarranted government intrusion

Physicians shudder when they see prospective lawmakers who

want to meddle in medical affairs. U.S. Senate candidate Todd Akin sank his 2012 campaign when he minimized the threat of pregnancy by rape.

"If it's a legitimate rape, the female body has ways to try to shut that whole thing down," said Akin, a Missouri Republican and former member of Congress.

Senate candidate Richard Mourdock, an Indiana Republican, did the same thing when he described pregnancies from rape as "something God intended to happen."

The American College of Physicians (ACP) finally had enough. It drafted guidelines aimed at legislators who are creating bills to regulate clinical decision-making. The principles seek to protect the doctor-patient relationship.

The document—called "Statement of Principles on the Role of Governments in Regulating the Patient-Physician Relationship"—opposes laws that supersede physicians' orders, establish mandates for specific health services and limitations on physician-patient discussions.

In a statement, ACP then-President Dr. David Bronson said, "Some recent laws and proposed legislation appear to inappropriately infringe on clinical medical practice and patient-physician relationships, crossing traditional boundaries and intruding into the realm of medical professionalism."

In other words, stay out of the exam room if you can't back it up with medical evidence. Don't tell us what to do or say.

The document cited several examples of state laws that are more about politics than medicine. For example, a Florida law prohibits physicians from asking questions about gun safety. Pediatricians especially consider guns a health issue because firearms are a leading cause of death and injury for young people.

Pennsylvania physicians can access trade-secret chemicals used in a natural-gas extraction method called fracking, but they are prohibited by law from discussing their findings with patients who may be suffering subsequent harm.

President Obama had to backtrack on an obscure provision of the ACA that barred physicians from asking patients about the presence of guns in the household. He signed an executive order in January 2013 to "clarify that the (ACA) does not prohibit doctors asking their patients about guns in their homes." The American Academy of Pediatrics had sent a strongly worded letter to the Obama administration saying that pediatric advocates "vehemently reject" the gun provision in the health-care law.

The provision was pushed by the National Rifle Association (NRA) toward the end of the ACA debate in 2010. It was unearthed in the wake of the December 2012 schoolhouse massacre of 20 children and six educators in Newtown, Conn.

NRA officials said they had requested the provision because they feared insurance companies could use such data to raise premiums on gun owners. However, physician groups and researchers suspected that the provision was part of a long-term strategy to foreclose federal support for studies of firearms violence.

Florida lawmakers in 2011 proposed jail time for physicians who asked about their patients' gun ownership. Gov. Rick Scott signed a watered-down version that required health-care workers to "refrain" from asking about firearms unless the providers believe "in good faith" that such information would be relevant. A federal judge in 2012 struck down the law as unconstitutional and blocked its enforcement. The ruling has been appealed.

Questions lawmakers should ask themselves

The American College of Physicians recommends that law-makers ask themselves the following questions when drafting health-care legislation, in order to weigh its appropriateness and potential impact on the physician-patient relationship.

- Is the content and information or care consistent with the best available medical evidence on clinical effectiveness and professional standards of care?
- Is the proposed law or regulation necessary to achieve public health objectives and, if so, is there any other reasonable way to achieve the same objectives?
- Could the presumed basis for a government role be better addressed through advisory clinical guidelines developed by professional societies?
- Does the content and information or care allow for flexibility based on individual patient circumstances and on the most appropriate time, setting and means of delivering such information or care?
- Is the proposed law or regulation required to achieve a public policy goal without preventing physicians from addressing the health care needs of individual patients?
- Does the content and information to be provided facilitate shared decision-making between patients and their physicians based on the best medical evidence and the physician's clinical judgment, or would it undermine shared decision-making?
- Is there a process for appeal to accommodate for specific circumstances or changes in medical standards of care?

Pleasing-the-patient imperative

Although patient relationships consistently rank at the top of physician-satisfaction surveys, that relationship is changing. Patients, their demands and time pressure are conspiring to sap physician autonomy.

According to consultant PwC, five trends are driving the transformation from patient encounter to "customer experience."

- **Increased cost sharing.** Higher deductibles and tiered pricing have forced patients to take a more active role in their health-care decisions.
- **The push for value by payers and the government.** There is a greater focus on cost containment, quality and transparency.
- **"On-demand" health care.** Nearly 1 out of 4 patients said they had sought treatment at a retail clinic in 2011.
- **Information access.** There is a decentralization of power as more patients seek health-care information on the Internet.
- **Health reform.** An estimated 30 million newly insured Americans will be seeking care, and standardized insurance means providers will have to differentiate themselves on the basis of customer service.

Physicians are being judged by new standards. The Institute of Medicine defined patient-centered care as taking into account patient preferences, needs and values. It is easy to confuse that with patient satisfaction, which has its roots in consumer marketing. Patient satisfaction, say physicians Joel Kupfer and Edward Bond, means the customer's expectations were met or exceeded. If not, the service is deemed low quality. Patient satisfaction is important, they say, because it means physicians are providing comfort, support and education. However, patient satisfaction and patient-centeredness differ, because physicians are not obligated to satisfy patients' demands in the latter.

Many physicians dislike the morphing of patients into "customers." Yet it is clear that the consumer-focused practices of other retail industries are seeping into the exam room. In an online survey of 6,000 consumers, PwC found that only 8 percent ranked price as the top factor in choosing a physician—despite the fact that it was the No. 1 priority for more than half the respondents in shopping for travel, health insurance or retail goods. Personal recommendations were more than twice as likely to influence the purchase of health-care services as any other consumer purchase. Nine out of 10 said they would be willing to recommend a physician or hospital after a positive experience.

Millions of patients rely on physician ratings websites such as Healthgrades.com, Vitals.com and Rate MDs.com. Half of Americans go on line to research health information, and about 40 percent use websites that review physicians.

However, each rating is based on an average of only 2.4 patients. That means one disgruntled patient can skew the ratings significantly. There is no significant difference in median number of reviews based on gender, city size or U.S. region.

Picking a physician is not like buying a commodity. Physician services clearly defy simple ratings. However, that does not stop those who try to provide them. Consumer Reports rated 487 Massachusetts primary care and pediatric practices in its July 2012 edition, assigning scores from one to four in each of five categories related to patient experience.

The state's physicians seemed to be comfortable with the

ratings' methodology. They were based on surveys completed by more than 64,000 adults, and ratings had to reach a statistically reliable level threshold for an individual physician to be included.

Even with anonymity, raters tend to give their physicians rave reviews. A study examined more than 386,000 physician ratings posted on the RateMDs.com website between 2005 and 2010. Begun in 2004, the website has the most user-submitted reviews. About 250,000 U.S. doctors have been rated at least once on the site, according to RateMDs.com co-founder John Swapceinski.

RateMDs.com assigns physicians an overall rating of one to five based on patient assessments of their knowledge and help-fulness. Physicians received an average quality rating of 3.93 out of five. Nearly half received a perfect five rating.

Consumers are not particularly adept at figuring out what excellent care is. In a study of breast-cancer patients, 55 percent said they had received "excellent" care—even though 88 percent got treatment that was consistent with the best-treatment guidelines.

Respondents seemed to be more focused on the treatment process—such as how well providers communicated, and the ease of service.

However, physician performance may not affect customer loyalty. In focus groups conducted for the Robert Wood Johnson Foundation, patients consistently said that they would not switch their physician even if the personal chemistry was poor.

What patients want most are well-trained physicians who offer easy access and spend time with them in exam rooms. These qualitative factors are much more prevalent in health care than in other consumer settings.

Many doctors already have trouble turning down patient requests. More than one out of three say they would yield to a patient who asks for a clinically unwarranted magnetic resonance imaging exam.

In October 2013, the Centers for Medicare and Medicaid Services (CMS) began withholding 1 percent of hospital reimbursement to be redistributed as incentives to the hospitals with the highest performance-measure scores. Patient-satisfaction metrics account for 30 percent of the score. The percentage of reimbursement withheld will rise to 2 percent in 2017.

Evidence indicates that physicians—especially those employed by hospital systems—have been altering the way they practice to please the patient.

Consider these results from an *Emergency Physicians Monthly* survey:

- More than 16 percent of medical professionals had their employment threatened by low patient satisfaction scores.
- 48 percent of providers said they altered medical treatment because of the potential for a negative report on a patient satisfaction survey, with 10 percent of those admitting they provided medically unnecessary care.
- In a South Carolina Medical Association survey, more than half of physicians said they had ordered tests they considered inappropriate, and nearly half said they had improperly prescribed antibiotics or narcotic pain medication, because of patient satisfaction surveys.

Nearly two out of three hospitals, health systems and large physician groups have annual incentive plans for doctors that include patient-satisfaction metrics as a factor, up from 43 percent in 2010.

A team of University of California at Davis researchers found that people who are the most satisfied with their doctors are more likely to be hospitalized, accumulate more health-care and drug expenditures, and have higher death rates than patients who are less satisfied with their care. The researchers speculated that the higher death rates were a result of patients putting themselves in harm's way more often because of excess treatment.

"Patient satisfaction is a widely emphasized indicator of health-care quality, but our study calls into question whether increased patient satisfaction, as currently measured and used, is a wise goal in and of itself," Joshua Fenton, associate professor in the UC Davis Department of Family and Community Medicine and lead author of the study, said in a statement.

"Doctors may order requested tests or treatments to satisfy patients rather than out of medical necessity, which may expose patients to risks without benefits," he said. "A better approach is to explain carefully why a test or treatment isn't needed, but that takes time, which is in short supply during primary-care visits."

In an editorial accompanying the UC-Davis study in the *Archives of Internal Medicine*, Dr. Brenda Sirovich wrote, "Numerous studies have found that patients are consistently highly satisfied with one of the most common downsides of medical care—false-positive test results and the downstream events that follow. Almost any unnecessary or discretionary test has a good chance of detecting an abnormality."

She wrote, "The direct relationship between customer satisfaction and subsequent consumption is doctrine in commerce and business. 'The customer is always right,' a phrase likely coined by Marshall Field, the department store magnate, in the late 19th century, is a credo that we, as consumers, may wish we encountered more often. Is health care any different? Apparently not."

Treatment guidelines and lack of time

The administrative burden on today's physician practice, coupled with increasing medical complexity, inevitably spills over into patient care. For every 100 Medicare patients, a typical primary-care physician interacts with 99 other doctors in 53 practices. The chance that a primary-care visit will result in a referral nearly doubled between 1999 and 2009.

About half of physicians say that they feel time pressure during office visits and that their work pace can be chaotic. More than three out of four feel they have little control over their work.

The frenetic pace of most physician offices is often characterized as hamster-wheel activity designed to maximize revenue. Physicians need to diagnose and treat quickly. Hasty diagnoses can lead to errors.

Best Doctors is a Boston-based health-care organization that treats 20 million people in 30 countries, essentially providing second opinions for large employers and insurance plans. It estimates that it changes the diagnosis in about 20 percent of the cases it reviews, and changes treatment in more than 60 percent of cases.

Job satisfaction among physicians is strongly tied to their relationships with patients. Those ties have been frayed by time and productivity pressures and administrative burdens. Physicians' sense of little control have fueled this disconnect—and discontent.

Attempting to keep up with voluminous—and sometimes conflicting—practice guidelines and peer-reviewed literature is nearly impossible. A group of researchers attempted to gauge the amount of effort required to keep up with primary-care research. They found 341 active journals with 8,265 articles in one month. They estimated that physicians would need 627 hours a month—nearly 21 hours a day—to evaluate the literature.

The Cochrane Collaboration created 1,837 systematic reviews addressing intervention-related questions and more than 11,600 abstracts of additional systematic reviews. That is barely scratching the surface. Cochrane personnel estimated it would take 30 years to summarize the existing controlled trials for Cochrane reviews—excluding the new evidence published during those 30 years.

Nine prominent physician groups have created a list of 45 frequently prescribed tests and treatments they say are often unnecessary and may even be harmful.

Each group, representing both primary-care doctors and specialists, picked five procedures that medical evidence shows have little or no value, and that they say should be questioned automatically by patients and their doctors.

Dr. David Sackett, a pioneer in evidence-based practice, said the effort integrates three important components: clinical expertise, a patient's values and preferences, and the best research available.

The problem is the third component. Two Welsh medical school professors appraised the "avalanche of information" heaped upon clinicians. They calculated that medical students training in cardiac imaging would need to read 40 papers every weekday for 11 years to become current with the specialty.

A chief reason many doctors cannot meet national clinical-care guidelines is a lack of time. A physician with a 2,500-patient panel would need 21.7 hours a day to meet recommended national clinical-care guidelines.

There are several barriers to adopting medical evidence as the standard for treatment, including the difficulty of changing physician practice patterns and the sheer volume of research. Translating science into medical practice takes an average of 17 years from discovery into practice, and monitoring the more than 10,000 randomized, controlled trials published annually is impossible for a busy clinician.

The research findings also change at a dizzying pace. An *Archives of Internal Medicine* study found that 13 percent of research articles published in the *New England Journal of Medicine* in 2009 were reversals of earlier research findings about prescription medications, screening tests and procedures.

A *JAMA* article examined studies that had found a particular medical practice effective. One-third were later followed by trials that found those practices either ineffective or less effective than originally reported.

Mayo Clinic Proceedings researchers examined articles from 2001 to 2010 in *The New England Journal of Medicine* and found 363 studies that tested a medical practice constituting the standard of care at the time. The published articles contradicted the established medical practice 40 percent of the time, adding up to 146 cases in which new evidence questioned the care physicians had been advised to provide.

Time constraints place even more pressure on physician-patient communication. Patients add to the burden by not taking care of their own health or demanding care that is inappropriate.

Patient participation in care decisions scarcely existed until 1960. Physicians were expected to promote patient welfare without necessarily acknowledging patient rights. Shared decision-making has been fueled by readily available information on the Internet and by consumer-driven health plans. Physicians increasingly are being seen as expert advisers to patients who want their care preferences and values to be part of the treatment equation.

This desire for patient autonomy creates different pressures for physicians. Complex medical science is difficult for physicians to explain and patients to understand. Mutual frustration creates the default scenario in which physicians are not inclined to engage in long discussions of treatment pros and cons, and patients often want doctors to make decisions for them.

The average physician visit lasts 18 minutes. A patient is able to speak for an average of 23 seconds before the physician interrupts. One out of three parents reported spending less than 10 minutes with the clinician at their last well-child visit, compared with only one out of five who spent more than 20 minutes. In a landmark 1984 study, fewer than 1 out of 4 patients were allowed to express their needs completely without interruption.

Trying to have a meaningful discussion under these circumstances is difficult. Physicians often select treatments based on what they believe their patients would want, absent an actual conversation.

Patient satisfaction is directly tied to more time with the physician and less time in the waiting room. DrScore.com, a physician-rating website, analyzed 36,000 patient surveys. It found physicians were considered less caring when wait times were longer than 15 minutes and visits were less than 10 minutes.

Most physician offices are set up to deal with acute conditions. However, nearly half of Americans have at least one chronic condition, requiring complex care and often involving coordination with several clinical, occupational and social services. More than four out of 10 physicians function without non-physician staff that can work with chronic-disease patients, such as nurse case managers and social workers.

Researchers taped 34 physicians during more than 300 patient visits. They found that physicians spent an average of 1.3 minutes imparting important information about the patient's condition and treatment, and much of that was too technical for most patients to understand. The physicians in this study remembered things differently: They estimated that they had spent more than eight minutes communicating about the patient's care.

Physicians forget important information their patients give them from one visit to the next about one-third of the time.

About one out of three elderly adults said their physicians did not review their medications, even though adverse drug events lead to more than 177,000 emergency-department visits annually. About two out of three said their doctors or nurses did not ask whether they had fallen or give advice about tripping on carpets or stumbling on stairs. Falls account for more than two million injuries annually for people 65 and older.

About three out of five patients believe their doctors are rushing through exams, a proportion that has barely moved for three decades.

There has been improvement in some aspects of physician-patient relations over time. NPR took questions from a 1983 poll and asked them again. This time, respondents gave doctors higher ratings in some categories. About two out of three said doctors usually explained things well to them, compared with 49 percent in 1983. More said doctors are trying to hold down medical costs.

More time in the courtroom than classroom

Medical malpractice suits are time-consuming and emotionally draining. The average physician spends more time—about 11 percent of his or her career—embroiled in malpractice litigation than it takes to complete medical school.

Most claims consume two years prior to resolution, and nearly twice that much time elapses since the event in question.

The defensive medicine practiced by health professionals to avoid lawsuits costs an estimated $60 billion annually, based on a survey of more than 1,200 physicians. That does not include the cost of carrying liability insurance. Many say the cost of defending—and avoiding—medical liability suits is siphoning funds away from needed health-care delivery reforms and infrastructure expenditures.

Consultant PwC, relying on that CBO report, estimated that malpractice insurance and defensive medicine accounted for 10 percent of total health-care costs. A 2010 *Health Affairs* article more conservatively pegged those costs at 2.4 percent of health-care spending.

In a 2010 survey, U.S. orthopedic surgeons bluntly admitted that about 30 percent of tests and referrals were medically unnecessary and done to reduce physician vulnerability to lawsuits.

Whether a physician practices defensive medicine may depend more on a doctor's fear of being sued than the level of pain-and-suffering damage caps and insurance premiums in that physician's state. Researchers surveyed physicians about their medical liability fears and examined their Medicare claims from 2007 to 2009. The more worried physicians were about litigation, the more likely they ordered more tests and advanced imaging, referred patients to an emergency department or admitted them to a hospital. The study suggests reformers should address physicians' fears more than limits on liability damages.

A 2011 analysis by the American Medical Association (AMA found that the average amount to defend a lawsuit in 2010 was $47,158, compared with $28,981 in 2001. The average cost to pay a medical liability claim—whether it was a settlement, jury award or some other disposition—was $331,947, compared with $297,682 in 2001.

Doctors spend significant time fighting lawsuits, regardless of outcome. The average litigated claim lingered for 25 months. Doctors spent 20 months defending cases that were ultimately dismissed, while claims going to trial took 39 months. Doctors who were victorious in court spent an average of 44 months in litigation.

Most physicians are sued at least once during their careers, and usually prevail. The frequency of medical liability claims varies by specialty. Neurosurgeons are sued the most—nearly 20 percent are defendants in a given year.

A study in *The New England Journal of Medicine* estimated that by age 65 about 75 percent of physicians in low-risk specialties have been the target of at least one lawsuit, compared with about 99 percent of those in high-risk specialties.

Nearly one out of four surgeons are engaged in litigation at any given time, according to a 2011 study. Those embroiled in lawsuits are more likely to suffer burnout, depression, emotional exhaustion and detachment, lower self-esteem or even suicidal thoughts.

The annual risk that physicians will be sued is about 5 percent in low-risk specialties, such as psychiatry and pediatrics, with a cumulative career risk of about 75 percent. In high-risk specialties such as neurosurgery and cardiac surgery, the annual risk is about 20 percent and cumulative career risk is 99 percent. In a welcome development for physicians, nearly 60 percent of medical liability premiums held steady in 2012, and about 26 percent decreased, according to the Medical Liability Monitor annual survey.

According to Brian Atchinson, president of the Physician Insurers Association of America (PIAA), 70 percent of legal claims do not result in payments to patients, and physician defendants prevail 80 percent of time in claims resolved by verdict.

The number and total value of physician malpractice payments dropped in 2011 for the eighth consecutive year. The 9,758 payments totaled $3.2 billion in 2011, which represents about .12 percent of total health-care costs.

Studies have found modest effects of prospective malpractice reform. A CBO report estimated that a package of five malpractice reforms would reduce national health spending by about 0.5 percent. A 2010 *Health Affairs* study calculated that a 10 percent decline in medical malpractice premiums would result in less than 1 percent of total health-care savings. That is because medical malpractice insurance accounts for less than 2 percent of national health spending.

However, those costs are significant to physicians. Texas placed limits on malpractice damages in 2003. Liability premiums fell from about $17,000 that year to about $10,300 in 2011 for family physicians. Rates fell from more than $48,000 to about $30,500 for general surgeons and from $53,800 to $33,900 for obstetrics and gynecology.

The Charter on Medical Professionalism sets standards on physician honesty and openness with patients. The document has been endorsed by more than 100 professional groups and the Accreditation Council for Graduate Medical Education.

Owning up to mistakes

A 2012 *Health Affairs* study tested those standards in a survey of about 1,900 physicians. About one out of 10 admitted that they had lied to a patient in the previous year. About one out of three did not agree that it is important to tell patients about their relationships with pharmaceutical or medical device companies. Two out of three said they agreed that physicians should disclose medical errors to patients. However, one out of five admitted that they had not disclosed a particular error in the past year, out of fear of being sued.

One out of three physicians do not agree that there is a need to tell affected patients about serious medical errors. However, fully informing them can defuse anger and lessen the likelihood that they will sue, according to a landmark 1999 *Annals of Internal Medicine* study. Some physicians specifically are reluctant to treat low-income patients because they fear potential litigation. For example, about half of California physicians who refused to treat uninsured or Medicaid patients cited what they perceived to be a heightened risk of being sued. However, studies show poor people are less likely to sue physicians, because of limited access to legal resources and a medical malpractice payment system that requires advance funding to litigate cases.

Physicians' malpractice concerns are the same regardless of whether they live in states that have adopted medical malpractice reforms. The fact that doctors almost inevitably will be defendants reflects the grip malpractice litigation has on the health-care system.

Some health-policy analysts have suggested giving clinicians "safe harbor" protection from liability when they follow clinical-practice guidelines. Doing so could be a triple win: better quality, reduction in costly defensive medicine and potentially a compromise in the long-standing partisan battle over tort-reform caps on awards. The unsuccessful 2009 Healthy Americans Act wanted clinical guidelines to serve as "rebuttable presumptions" that care was not negligent.

However, the proliferation of often-conflicting guidelines makes it difficult to settle on any given one. "Safe harbor" also assumes unrealistically that there is conclusive evidence of what exactly is appropriate care in a given situation.

Dr. David Hyman and Charles Silver argued in the journal *Chest* that five myths persist about medical malpractice:

- Malpractice crises are caused by spikes in payouts and claim frequency.
- The tort system yields "jackpot justice."
- One verdict can bankrupt a physician.
- Physicians move to states that have damage caps.
- Tort reform would lower health-care spending significantly.

They said payouts per physician have been declining since 2003 and are now nearly half of the 1992 level. They said only about 2 percent of cases go to trial, and providers win about three out of four cases. They said only physicians "who grossly underinsure" themselves place their personal assets at risk after losing a case.

Regardless, the authors acknowledged the medical malpractice process was expensive, slow and "perceived by everyone involved" as difficult and "often unjust and unfair."

CHAPTER 9

Everything But Patient Care

What happened to Eastern Carolina internal Medicine (ECIM) in Pollocksville, N.C., is a provider's nightmare about government oversight run amok.

A Medicare audit began as a medical records request. The auditor alleged minor errors in the medical charts and then extrapolated an overpayment amount. A demand for $40,000 in alleged over payments from Medicare quickly escalated to more than $1 million. To be paid immediately.

"The federal government said to us, 'You are a crook. You've overcharged. You owe us this amount of money," said practice founder Dr. Neil Bender.

After two years of fighting the charges, ECIM prevailed. To achieve the victory, ECIM physicians and staff reviewed each questioned claim in court, which consumed three days. An administrative law judge ruled that ECIM documentation was correct on more than 90 percent of the disputed claims, and lowered the fine to just over $3,500. The defense cost $300,000 in legal and other fees, thousands of hours of lost patient care, and interest paid on $700,000 the practice had borrowed to pay the alleged CMS fine up to that point.

Dr. Robert Monteiro, an ECIM internist, said the payments were "tantamount to paying a full practice partner who does not bring in any revenue. It killed cash flow and put us in a tough position. The event was extremely traumatic."

Even after the ruling, CMS continued to demand payments until ECIM supplied the agency with a copy of the judge's ruling. The practice required the intervention of Sen. Richard Burr, R-N.C., to recover the unwarranted payments it had already made to the government. The interest that the government paid back on those funds was less than the interest rate the practice had paid on the initial loan.

Monteiro said ECIM was not an isolated case. He said he had heard of other North Carolina practices that received the same harsh treatment.

"Some gave up and paid, some closed their practices, and others fought like we did," he said.

Monteiro said the financial stress of the audit fight eventually led to ECIM's selling its practice to CarolinaEast Medical Center in nearby New Bern. It became CarolinaEast Internal Medicine.

"What happened to this rural North Carolina medical practice is unacceptable," Burr said. "While oversight systems can play an appropriate role in helping to root out fraud and waste, it should be done in a consistent and predictable process to ensure medical practices such as ECIM are not inappropriately targeted and unfairly burdened in the future."

The North Carolina Medical Society produced a documentary about the saga, *Guilty Until Proven Innocent: When Medicare*

Audits Cause Casualties.

"This documentary offers an example of the real-life consequences of a federal government audit program that is out of control," said Robert Seligson, executive vice president and CEO of the medical society.

Suburban Dallas rheumatologist Dr. Fehmida Zahabi was exasperated.

She found herself surrounded by 21 prior-authorization requests for various treatments and medications. Insurance companies, she said, have made a seemingly simple process complicated.

Zahabi, co-director of the Rheumatology Society of North Texas, said nearly 70 percent of physicians have difficulty figuring out which medicines a patient's insurance company covers and which medications require prior authorization. On the other hand, an insurance company has no time limit to decide whether to pay for the medication.

In Texas, health insurance companies had 258 different pre-authorization forms for prescribed medications prior to reforms passed by the 2013 Texas legislature.

Zahabi estimates she spends 15 to 20 percent of her office time on pre-authorizations.

"I have people to do the logistics, but I have to do the clinical aspects and it has to have my signature for legitimacy. The wording (on the forms) is not good English and has double negatives. It's a brainless activity, but it's like taking a test. It's pathetic.

"They (insurance companies) want the exact dates that a patient has been using a medication. If they stopped, they want to know when and why. Imagine a patient who has been transferred to my care. Where do I get this piece of information? This is onerous. They make you feel like you are a fifth-grade kid making decisions capriciously. Doesn't make sense."

Credentialing and other systems for provider contracts with health plans are rife with redundancy. Many organizations collect virtually identical information. The typical physician spends more than three hours a year submitting nearly 18 different credentialing forms—many of which are nearly the same— with staff spending an additional 20 hours. A coordinated nationwide credentialing system could save providers nearly $1 billion annually. Standardized electronic payer-provider contracts could achieve further savings.

Long waits for insurance authorization allowing psychiatric patients to be admitted to the hospital from the emergency department waste thousands of hours of physician time, given that most such requests are ultimately granted. A commentary in *Annals of Emergency Medicine* argued that the pre-authorization process is akin to health care "rationing by hassle factor."

U.S. physicians have been called the most "second-guessed and paperwork-laden physicians in western industrialized democracies."

Doctors' workdays

According to a 2010 American Medical Association (AMA) survey, a typical physician office spends 20 hours a week on insurance administrative tasks. It found that more than two out of three physicians typically wait several days for pre-authorization for medications and one out of 10 wait more than a week. A 2009 *Health Affairs* study found that interactions with insurance companies cost U.S. physicians $23.2 billion to $31 billion a

THE BURDEN OF PAPERWORK

Q: How many hours do you work each week on non-clinical (paperwork) duties only?

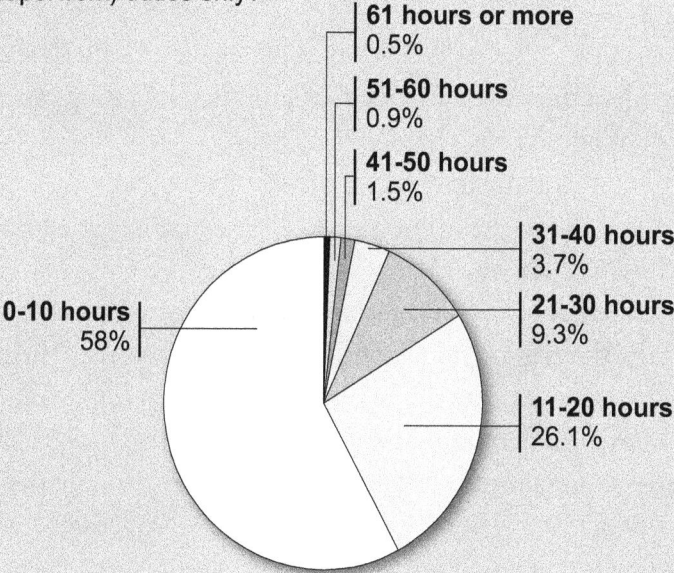

61 hours or more
0.5%

51-60 hours
0.9%

41-50 hours
1.5%

31-40 hours
3.7%

0-10 hours
58%

21-30 hours
9.3%

11-20 hours
26.1%

Source: Physicians Foundation Survey of America's Physicians, 2012.

More than 4 out of 10 physicians spend at least 10 hours a week on non-clinical duties.

year.

The average physician spends nearly three weeks per year dealing with health plans. In addition, 23 weeks of nursing staff time and 44 weeks of clerical staff time are spent on insurance claims.

Physicians spend 45 percent of their workday outside the exam room, much of it devoted to documentation and follow-up. Every minute a physician spends outside direct patient care costs the average practice $4 to $6 in lost revenue.

With the widespread use of electronic health records (EHR), *Health Affairs* researchers estimated that at least half of a physician's time during a patient visit is spent on low-value clerical work.

Dr. Alan Plummer, professor of medicine at Emory University, said all of the Physicians Foundation watch issues are important, but administrative burdens stand out.

"They all sort of interact," he said. "They overburden the doctor and create less time to see each patient. Or (doctors) take the same amount of time and see fewer patients. That cuts down the productivity. If they have to do 10 minutes extra to do the EHR, that's going to take time from everyone else," he said.

Don Alexander, former chief executive officer of the Tennessee Medical Association, said , "Doctors say, 'If you place more burdens on my practice, I have less time with my patients and see fewer of them. Then I have to raise fees to cover my costs,' " he said.

Gary Price, a plastic surgeon in Guilford, Conn., said, "The regulatory burden continues to get worse and worse. It's death by a thousand cuts. I only do surgery on healthy people. I'm required to have them sign a form on whether they have living wills. Admittedly, it only takes four or five minutes to deal with, but I have hundreds of these kinds of things. I have electronic health records, and that does not make it quicker. These things constantly irritate doctors," he said.

Dr. Joseph Valenti, an obstetrician and gynecologist in Denton, Texas, said the biggest obstacle to practicing medicine is the administrative burden.

"It's really starting to get in the way. But doctors are trying to see more patients to make up for less reimbursement. Patients want us to spend time with them. We want to spend time with them. Yet we are spending more time on things that don't add to patient care," he said.

Valenti estimates he spends about 20 percent of his time on administrative tasks, but has spoken to other physicians who say they spend 40 to 50 percent of theirs "documenting and jumping through hoops" to get paid.

Valenti said government insurance reimbursement is so low, the administrative burden feels heavier. He said Medicaid in Texas pays about 68 percent of Medicare rates and about 60 percent of private insurance rates.

For Medicaid, he said, "you can't do certain things without clearance. They harass us about this and that. It's troublesome, because we know how to take care of our patients."

Managed care tactics from the 1990s return

Insurance companies have been employing tactics reminiscent of managed care in the 1990s, according to *The Wall Street Journal*. They subtly are erecting more barriers to care through tighter networks and by requiring more referrals and authorizations prior to care.

In 2012, the AMA found a 23 percent increase over 2011 in claims that reflected an insurer pre-authorization review—increasing the total to 4.7 percent of claims. The AMA estimated that prior authorization policies added $728 million in administrative costs in 2012.

Doctors must follow strict health-plan guidelines or they will not be reimbursed. State and federal health-insurance programs continue to squeeze the rates they pay physicians. Many practices lose money when they treat Medicaid and Medicare patients.

Physicians have to hustle to cover their costs. Laurie Green, a San Francisco obstetrician and gynecologist, told the *Journal*, "I live my life in seven-minute intervals." She estimated that she needed to earn $70 every 15 minutes to cover her office overhead.

Physicians' workdays generally are brutal. A Philadelphia practice kept track of what its physicians did in a day's time. The average doctor saw 18 patients, wrote 12 prescriptions, reviewed 14 consultation reports from specialists, studied 11 X-rays or other imaging reports, and wrote or answered 17 emails.

Of the time physicians spend outside of office visits, about one-third was spent on activities that saved an average of five visits a day, such as telephone calls and email communication with patients. The good news is that these activities reduce health-care costs, save time for patients and improve care co-ordination. The bad news for physicians is that these activities usually are not reimbursed.

Primary care, especially, is larded with unpaid work. An *Archives of Internal Medicine* study found that a typical general internist's day included 70 laboratory tests, images and consultations; writing or signing 31 prescriptions; responding to seven messages related to patient care; and reviewing, editing and signing 17 electronic health records. This work is largely invisible and off the clock. Such administrative tasks add to an already crushing workload and can hasten physician burnout.

According to a 2013 physician survey by Medscape, nearly 40 percent reported at least one symptom of burnout, such as emotional exhaustion and a diminished sense of accomplishment. The top two reasons were "too many bureaucratic tasks" and "spending too many hours at work."

ADMINISTRATIVE BURDEN

Q: Why is the profession in decline?

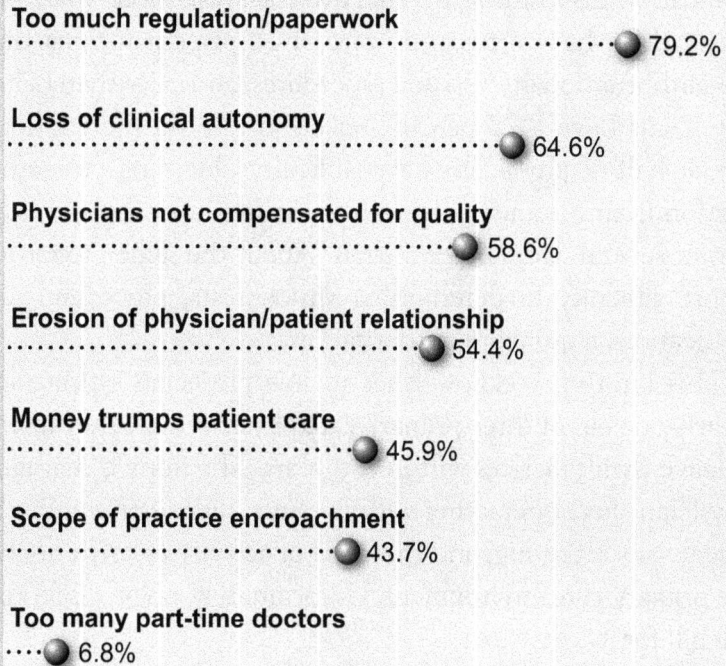

Too much regulation/paperwork
....● 79.2%

Loss of clinical autonomy
....● 64.6%

Physicians not compensated for quality
....● 58.6%

Erosion of physician/patient relationship
....● 54.4%

Money trumps patient care
...............................● 45.9%

Scope of practice encroachment
............................● 43.7%

Too many part-time doctors
....● 6.8%

Source: Physicians Foundation Survey of America's Physicians, 2012.

Nearly 8 out of 10 physicians say the profession is declining because of administrative burden.

Many health systems unwittingly are pushing more work onto the physician because they fear violating institutional or federal compliance issues. In some cases, only the physician can turn on the computer, reconcile a patient's medications, record the history, enter orders for tests, compose the after-visit summary and complete the billing invoice—tasks that could be done by other staff members.

More than three out of four physicians believe insurers demand excessive pre-authorization for tests, procedures and medications, according to an AMA survey. More than one out of three have a rejection rate of 20 percent for first-time pre-authorization on tests and procedures, and more than half of physicians have a 20 percent rejection rate on prescriptions. About half of physicians have difficulty obtaining pre-authorization from insurance plans. About two out of three typically wait several days for permission. About the same proportion report difficulty in determining which tests, procedures and medications require pre-authorization.

This kind of workflow leads to low physician satisfaction. Nearly one out of three primary-care physicians say they intend to leave their practices within two years. The irony is that most physicians find interacting with patients outside of reimbursed office visits satisfying, and this kind of activity clearly enriches the primary-care environment. Unfortunately, no one is footing the bill for it.

Providers are attempting to push back against administrative burdens by becoming more efficient in other areas. Two process-improvement methodologies, such as Lean and Six Sigma, have migrated from other industries into health care.

Lean focuses on eliminating waste, such as excessive motion, excessive wait times and unnecessary processing. Six Sigma attempts to reduce variation in activity. Examples include checklists for evidence-based activities and flowcharts to identify tasks that benefit both physician and patient.

Lack of productivity

The health-care sector is expected to grow by 23 percent—or about three million new jobs—between 2008 and 2018, compared with 9 percent for all other employment sectors.

The number of jobs in physician offices is expected to rise by about one-third this decade, to about three million employees. The rate of growth of jobs in hospitals will be half of that. Physician-office employment rose 2.8 percent in 2011, or by about 65,000 jobs.

Unfortunately, not all of this job growth is translating into more productivity. One study found that labor productivity in physician practices between 1990 and 2010 actually fell 0.6 percent. The decline in output was measured as the number of physician visits, tests, treatment and surgeries per unit of cost.

The study underscores the administrative bloat that pervades health care. Simply moving money from the payer to the provider based on negotiated rates is extremely expensive. Billing and insurance-related functions can account for more than half of administrative expenses at a hospital or large physician practice. For an insurance company, the share can exceed 80 percent.

Harvard Business Review researchers calculated that the health-care workforce grew by 75 percent from 1990 to 2012. Of that, only 5 percent were physicians. The ratio of physicians to non-physician workers is 1:16. Of those 16, 10 are administrative and management staff, with the balance being mid-level clinicians.

Despite the erosion of health-care reimbursement, more than half of the 50 U.S. jobs that are projected to grow the fastest from 2013 to 2017 are in health care.

The insurance bureaucracy

The U.S. spends about three times as much on health-care administration and insurance per capita as Canada. Brookings Institution economist Henry Aaron estimated in 2003 that the U.S. would save more than $213 billion annually in administration and insurance costs if it had a single-payer system similar to that nation's.

In fact, the entire health-care system is inflated with costly administrative tasks. According to the Institute of Medicine (IOM), the United States spends $361 billion annually on health-care administration—double the treatment costs of heart disease and triple the cost of cancer. The IOM estimates half of these expenditures are unnecessary.

Aaron described the U.S. health-care system as "an administrative monstrosity, a truly bizarre mélange of thousands of payers with payment systems that differ for no socially beneficial reason, as well as staggeringly complex public systems with mind-boggling administered prices and other rules expressing distinctions that can only be regarded as weird."

Donald Berwick, former director of the Centers for Medicare and Medicaid Services, estimated that needless administrative complexity created $107 billion to $389 billion in wasteful health-system spending in 2011. He cited "government, accreditation agencies, payers and others (who) create inefficient and misguided rules. For example, payers may fail to standardize forms, thereby consuming limited physician time in needlessly complex billing procedures."

For example, Johns Hopkins Health System in Baltimore deals with about 700 different health plans, employers and other payers. Each payer has an annually negotiated rate for each service. Each also has different payment cycles and eligibility rules that must be tracked. The sheer complexity creates its own redundancies in several Johns Hopkins departments, which the organization calculated to be more than $40 million annually.

According to a study by a University of Massachusetts professor, a single-payer system would save the U.S. $1.8 trillion over a decade—including $592 billion in 2014 alone. Those savings would stem from eliminating the administrative burden of the current system and using the government's bargaining power to drive down the cost of pharmaceuticals.

According to a 2008 study, 59 percent of U.S. physicians support a single-payer system. That is no doubt a measure of the enormous frustration physicians feel toward the nation's insurance bureaucracy. In a 2011 survey of physicians who said they were "moderately to severely stressed or burned out on an average day," the leading cause cited was the administrative demands of the job.

The AMA has been leading an effort to cut in half the number of medical claims paid incorrectly by large insurers.

The percentage of claims incorrectly processed by health plans fell for the third straight year, to about 7 percent, in 2013, according to the AMA's sixth National Health Insurer Report Card. That compares with a 2011 rate of more than 19 percent. The AMA estimated that more than $43 billion could have been saved if commercial insurers had paid all claims correctly since 2010.

The AMA created an Administrative Burden Index to rank insurers based on unnecessary costs. The index rates commercial plans using a "star rating" based on delayed remittance, prior authorization requirements, claim edits and claim denials.

According to its fifth annual National Health Insurer Report Card, error rates for private health insurers on paid medical claims dropped from 19.3 percent in 2011 to 9.5 percent in 2012. This improvement resulted in $8 billion in health system savings, because of the reduction in unnecessary administrative work to reconcile errors. While dramatic improvements were made in 2013, the commercial health-insurance industry still paid the wrong amount for nearly one out of 14 medical claims.

Government is the bigger villain

Insurance companies used to be the prime source of administrative burden. They have been supplanted by government, according to physicians and their advocates.

"It used to be the insurance companies (that imposed more burden), but commercial insurers are trying to make things simpler. With the government, there's meaningful use, HIPAA, PQRS, ICD-10...the list goes on and on," said Louis Goodman, Texas Medical Association chief executive officer and president of the Physicians Foundation

Robert Seligson, chief executive officer of the North Carolina Medical Society, quipped, "What insurance misses (in administrative burden), the government makes sure it fills the void."

Todd Atwater, chief executive officer of the South Carolina Medical Association and a member of the South Carolina state legislature, said his association and MGMA have funded a grant to identify specific physician administrative burdens that they can reduce.

Atwater said insurance companies were the focus a few years ago, but physicians have gotten used to the game and learned

COMPARISON WITH OTHER INDUSTRIES

Estimate of billing- and insurance-related employees in the health care enterprise and comparison with other industries.

Revenue cycle FTEs per $1 billion revenue

	0	200	400	600	800
Health care services					●
Consumer products	●				
Industrial goods	●				
Other service providers	●				
All industries	●				

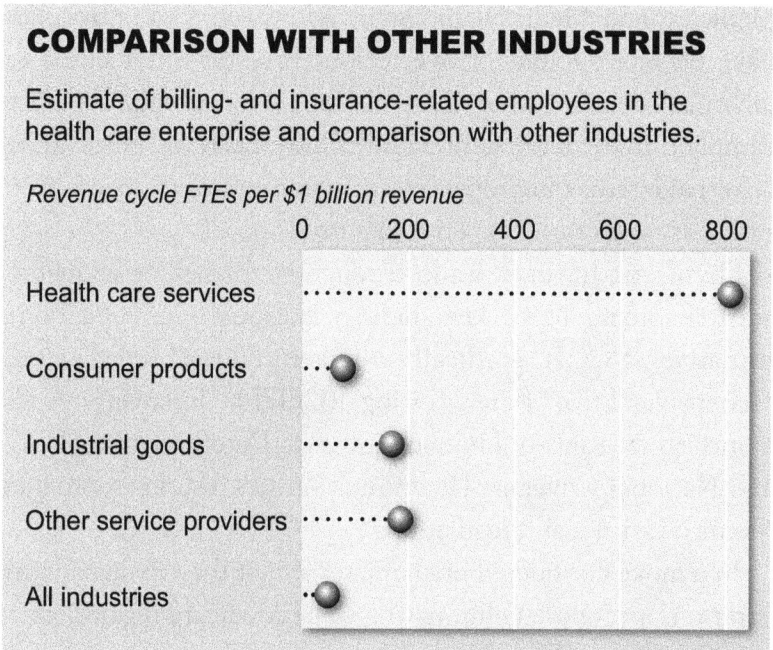

Source: Moses, et al. JAMA. 2013;310(18).

Compared with other industries, health care has many times more employees devoted to billing and collections

to live with the hassle. The ACA imposes a new set of burdens, and physicians are trying to get in front of them.

Four of the top five financial challenges facing physician practices are government-related, according to a survey by CareCloud and Quantia MD. The top challenge is declining reimbursements, which physicians blamed largely on government insurance programs. They also point to ACA reporting and care requirements, coding and documentation changes, including ICD-10, and costs related to adoption of electronic health records.

CMS has been aggressive in pursuing fraud and abuse in

Medicare and Medicaid programs. However, some physicians have become victims of overzealous investigators focused on technical details rather than obvious wrongdoing. Providers complain that government auditors have been too quick to declare paid claims improper, requiring providers to spend up to two years and untold expense to pursue appeals.

Physicians have to wade through a thicket of audit-program acronyms to be law-abiding: National Correct Coding Initiative (NCCI), Medically Unlikely Edits (MUEs), Comprehensive Error Rate Testing (CERT), Recovery Audit Contractors (RACs), Limited Coverage Determination (LCD) and National Coverage Determination (NCD). Each program has its own rules and regulations.

In a move considered uncharacteristic of the Obama administration, it proposed eliminating some Medicare regulations, a move that it said would save hospitals and other health-care providers an estimated $676 million annually.

"We are committed to cutting the red tape for health-care facilities, including rural providers. By eliminating outdated or overly burdensome requirements, hospitals and health-care professionals can focus on treating patients," Health and Human Services Secretary Kathleen Sebelius said in a statement.

However, unfunded Medicare mandates hamper already struggling physician practices with expenses and time-sapping tasks they can ill afford, regardless of how well-meaning the regulations. Medicare regulations take up 125,000 pages. If laid out vertically page by page, they would extend for more than 21 miles.

Physician practices have been required since 2000 to provide translators at $150 or more for Medicare and Medicaid patients not proficient in English. Medicare will not reimburse practices for that or other services required to communicate better with patients.

Physicians will be required to submit quality-reporting-system measures to CMS even after quality bonus payments end in 2014, or else be penalized. Paying the penalty may be cheaper than absorbing the reporting costs.

The ACA has come to symbolize government regulation at its worst. Congressional Republicans constructed a "Red Tape Tower" by printing every ACA regulation. The tower is a seven-foot, 300-pound stack of paper that is pushed on a dolly to congressional offices and committee hearing rooms as Exhibit A of Washington over-regulation. Republicans claim the estimated 20,000 pages comprise nearly 190 million paperwork-burden hours that will be borne by the health-care industry, according to the Obamacare Burden Tracker, a report compiled by House GOP committee staff.

Long-delayed ICD-10

Physicians got a reprieve when Congress voted on March 31, 2014, to delay implementation of ICD-10 at least until Oct. 1, 2015. The AMA and other medical societies had told the federal government that the complicated system, with its diagnostic and procedure codes, would interfere with the migration to electronic health records.

A December 2012 letter from those groups to then-acting CMS administrator Marilyn Tavenner stated, "Stopping the implementation of ICD-10 is a critical, necessary step for removing regulatory burdens on physicians and ensuring that small physician practices are able to keep their doors open."

The previous month, the AMA House of Delegates had approved official policy to urge the elimination of the ICD-10 mandate and reiterate to CMS, which is overseeing the transition, that the burdens imposed by it will force many physicians out of business.

ICD-10 has about 68,000 codes, a fivefold increase from ICD-9's roughly 13,000 codes, the letter pointed out. Internal billing systems, for example, would require upgrades, and staff will need training to familiarize themselves with the codes. The new system expands the codes to three to seven digits, compared with the current 3 to 5 digits.

ICD-10 opponents like to point to some of the more arcane codes, such as the three separate codes for squirrel bites and being burned by flaming water skis.

"Physicians will be responsible for all of these costs, which, depending on the size of a medical practice, will range from $83,290 to more than $2.7 million," the letter to Tavenner stated.

The letter pointed out that the added financial and administrative burden was onerous for physician practices that were striving to participate in Medicare-led quality programs and attain meaningful use of electronic health records.

CMS had remained steadfast on the new October 2014 implementation deadline. In a letter to the American Health Information Management Association, CMS said the one-year extension it granted provides ample time for providers and payers for training and system upgrades.

There are two salient points about the ICD-10 conversion. First, a Canadian study that examined dually coded hospital discharge data using both ICD-9 and ICD-10 found that the latter was not materially different from that of ICD-9. That means

ICD-10 was not a measurable improvement in coding clinical data. Second, ICD-11 is scheduled for 2016, just two years later. Many have suggested skipping the cost and hassle of installing and training for ICD-10 and instead waiting for its successor.

Rep. Ted Poe (R-Texas) mocked ICD-10 from the House floor, pointing out that its codebook lists nine separate ways to be injured by a turkey and three ways to be injured by a lamp-post.

"It's red tape, it's bureaucracy, and this is what happens when clueless big government here in Washington starts telling people out in the workplace—doctors and patients—what they must do, and when government intrudes into our lives with more regulations," Poe said.

One coding expert estimated that nearly 65 percent of clinical documentation lacks enough information for coders to use for billing under ICD-10. Another estimated that physicians would spend 4 to 11 percent more time at their practices because of the change.

CHAPTER 10

Thriving Amid the Chaos

N early 60 percent of independent physicians want to stay
that way, including two out of three solo practitioners.
They say they value their autonomy and long-term relationships with their patients.

It is beyond the scope of this book to examine in detail all
of the alternatives for physicians seeking to preserve their autonomy and remain financially independent. The following
vignettes offer glimpses of physicians who successfully have
pursued strategies to survive and thrive independently in the
quickly evolving delivery-reform landscape.

The consummate medical home

When Dr. John Bender gives a visitor a tour of Miramont
Family Medicine in Fort Collins, Colo., he is like a docent.
Each room seems to have its own script. He has given this tour
dozens of times.

Among his visitors are physicians who want to see how he
created a patient-centered medical home (PCMH). There are

policymakers who want to see how he has been able to cut costs and improve quality. Others marvel at his state-of-the-art electronic medical records (EMR).

Bender bought one of the oldest family practices in the city in 2002. The office setup, a throwback to the 1970s, consisted of one physician, one medical assistant (MA) and an IBM computer for billing.

Bender immediately discovered he had a customer-service nightmare on his hands. The turnaround on test results was slow. He had no open appointments for patient emergencies. The office wallowed in non-revenue-producing activity. He had illegible documentation and no digital clinical data. Marketplace competitors—retail and urgent-care clinics, emergency departments (EDs), other practices—were eating his lunch.

Over the next decade, he built the practice into a highly efficient primary-care empire. He doubled the size of his practice every two years, and consistently has been cited as one of the fastest-growing companies in northern Colorado.

Eight physicians, a nurse practitioner and four physician assistants now treat 27,000 patients in four Miramont locations. They are supported by 50 employees and more than 80 computer workstations networked into an integrated data center. Team-based care includes team huddles for pre-visit planning, registry reporting and review, care coordination and test tracking.

In 2008, the practice received Level 3 PCMH recognition from the National Committee for Quality Assurance. Two years later, it won the national Nicholas E. Davies Award of Excellence from the Healthcare Information and Management Systems Society for its EMR. The Colorado Academy of Family Physicians Foundation named Miramont the PCMH of the Year.

Miramont is part of one of the nation's most robust prima-ry-care pilot projects, called the Colorado Multi-Payer PCMH Pilot. The project includes 16 family medicine and internal medicine practices along the Colorado Front Range. Health-TeamWorks, previously known as the Colorado Clinical Guidelines Collaborative, coordinated the project.

Seven health plans—WellPoint, UnitedHealthcare, Huma-na, Aetna, Cigna, Colorado Medicaid and CoverColorado — also participate, agreeing to pay practices a per-member, per-month fee for up to 20,000 patients per practice. That money helped the practices establish and maintain activities such as care management and care coordination.

For Miramont, medical-home pilot incentives represent about $150,000 to $200,000 of its $4.5 million in annual revenue.

"We are still mostly a fee-for-service shop," Bender said. "We take phone calls and emails because we are a medical home, but we gravitate toward reimbursable activities. We try to come up with solutions to justify reimbursement. We have a laser focus on reducing waste and inefficiency."

The practice layout reflects that aspiration. The nurse station is back-to-back with the front counter to process patients more efficiently. Exam rooms are arrayed so that the physician can reach equipment and the computer terminal without taking a step. Bender called it "a production cell."

Specialists rent space within the clinic to see Bender's pa-tients. They also have access to his EMR.

"In the old days, I would spend 40 minutes with a depressed patient and maybe didn't do any good, and it messed up the schedule for the rest of the afternoon. Now they get 15 min-utes and an antidepressant. They will get three or four hours of counseling (by a specialist in his office) before I see them again. And I have 80 percent patient follow-through because the specialists are here. Before, I would be lucky if I had one out of five compliance," he said.

His specialist tenants include a psychologist, an audiologist, a physical therapist and an acupuncturist.

Bender also has loaded the office with ancillary services and broadened his practice to do testing, lab work and minor surgical procedures. He believes he is saving his patients time and spending health-care dollars wisely.

"We save the system millions. We haven't referred anyone to a dermatologist or plastic surgeon for years. We do as many things as possible that we used to send to specialists: allergy shots, cast boots, stress testing, spirometry," he said.

Bender said he can handle about 80 percent of lab work in-house and does HIV testing. He also has a small pharmacy, where a technician dispenses about 140 pharmaceutical products, 20 percent of which are $6 generics. He even stocks competitively priced aspirin, pregnancy tests, tobacco-cessation aids and Band-Aids.

The practice has extended office hours to 8 p.m. Monday through Friday, and 9 a.m. to noon on Saturday.

Miramont was able to have a financial impact on treatment of Medicaid patients. Its per-patient cost was $11,633 a year, which was below the state Medicaid average. More significantly, ED use was more than 200 percent below the state Medicaid average.

Bender believes that he has earned the pilot incentive payments and that the insurance companies can well afford it.

"The pilot doesn't cost them that much. For them to pay

primary-care physicians a little extra is a blip on their revenue screen," he said.

The pilot paid physicians in three ways. The standard fee-for-service is maintained because volume incentives motivate physicians to treat patients in order to keep them out of the ED and more expensive specialty care. Physicians are also paid a per-member, per-month fee to support non-revenue activities such as EMR, online patient portals and care coordinators. Finally, they are paid bonuses for performance quality.

The metrics are tabulated monthly, and then reported back to the practice alongside those of other pilot practices for comparison. Sharing data motivates physicians and practice staff to improve weak performance and sustain strong results. The best performers share their success strategies during quarterly day-long retreats and bimonthly conference calls. HealthTeam-Works also provides on-site coaches who meet weekly with clinic staff to teach work-flow strategy and design.

Encouraged by the data, payers decided to extend the pilot, which had been scheduled to end in April 2012. According to Bender, the pilot showed that health-care cost reductions more than offset the increased payments to physicians in the pilot, with break-even at between 12 and 24 months. He said PCMH work-flow changes are scalable to urban, suburban or rural practices within two years.

The medical village

Lauren Burch, a Plano, Texas, mother with two children, was visiting relatives in Lubbock. Her infant son, Owen, became ill and could not seem to shake a viral stomach illness. She emailed her physician, Dr. Sander Gothard of Village Health

Partners (VHP) in Plano. He sent back instructions to see a local physician and consulted with the Lubbock doctor about the child's medical background and clues as to what might be wrong. Burch says the email exchange averted potentially serious consequences.

Burch pays VHP $100 annually for unlimited email access to Gothard, and queries him about four times a month. Burch estimates these exchanges have prevented more than half of potential office visits. She says her husband doesn't like to go to the doctor and uses email whenever possible. About 5 percent of VHP's patients pay for the extra access.

Gothard and Dr. Christopher Crow are two of VHP's seven co-founders. Crow, the practice's public face, is an evangelist about making health care accessible, convenient and high quality. He has a master's degree in business administration and the outlook of an efficiency-minded executive. VHP was an early adopter of EMR, buying its first system in 2003. Crow estimates the $100,000 investment paid for itself in 18 months.

VHP has leveraged technology and standardized processes to reduce its support staff well below the national average. The average family practice employs 5.5 people to support each physician; VHP can do so with a ratio of less than 3.5 to 1.

Although VHP is recognized as a model medical home, Crow is much more enthusiastic about the practice's location: Legacy Medical Village. There, 23 medical specialty practices conveniently operate under one roof. Patients can see a doctor, fill prescriptions, get lab and imaging services, and even see a consulting surgeon in less than half a day without leaving the 100,000-square-foot facility. Crow calls this Health 2.0, where 95 percent of necessary care is at one location.

The success of VHP and Legacy Medical Village certainly raises the question: Why there are not more medical facilities such as these? Crow talks about the need for physicians to invest in EMR, assertively coordinate care, and have a passion for customer service.

Each day, the busy practice sees 250 patients and receives about 700 phone calls, 400 faxes and 100 emails. Phone calls are usually answered within 30 seconds. There is no voice mail or phone tree.

Crow estimates the MAs can handle 90 percent of phone inquiries from patients. They also use EMR to remind callers about preventive care.

"We have more than 1,000 opportunities a day to check for gaps in care," Crow says. "We organize our practice around those opportunities."

VHP's clinical quality metrics reflect the results. For example, its recommended breast-cancer screening rate is 79 percent, compared with the national average of 43 percent. It also exceeds national averages in colorectal cancer screening, smoking-cessation counseling and diabetes control.

The practice also monitors ED visits by its patients at local hospitals, proactively calling to help create discharge care plans. Crow says hospital emergency rooms rarely communicated with VHP about patient care prior to the monitoring.

VHP was named Practice of the Year by *Physicians Practice* magazine in 2006. The Healthcare Information and Management Systems Society named VHP the nation's most adept physician practice at using technology and medical records in 2007—three years before Miramont in Colorado. Its village concept has attracted visitors from the state legislature and U.S.

Congress; Crow also was asked to visit with Obama administration officials in Washington.

Crow has expanded his village concept to two other Plano locations, with a total of 30 providers treating more than 75,000 patients.

Medical village 2.0

Kevin Spencer, an Austin, Texas, family physician, also is creating a medical village. Spencer collaborated with Crow on how to do it, and Southwest Medical Village was scheduled to open in January 2014. The 18-acre, 80,000-square-foot facility houses a variety of health-care providers, and Spencer's Premier Family Physicians (PFP) is the anchor tenant. PFP grew from a practice of six physicians in 2006 and has had four mergers since the passage of the Affordable Care Act.

Spencer, who has 32 providers in four Austin locations, sees two layers of patient engagement: traditional patient contacts by phone or walk-ins, and digitally.

Spencer got rid of his voice-messaging system in 2012 and put MAs on the line to assist callers.

"People are calling for a reason," he said. "They need advice about whether to make an appointment. People need to be walked through that. We try to make that experience better. Every touch is an opportunity. We decided to put the humans up front. It is a very elementary way for people to feel cared for. That's the whole reason we're here."

Spencer maintains that there are 15 common reasons people call, and the MAs are trained to handle each reason. If the call does not pertain to any of those reasons, it is transferred to a clinical provider.

KEEPING THE PRACTICE

Most physician practice owners want to stay independent

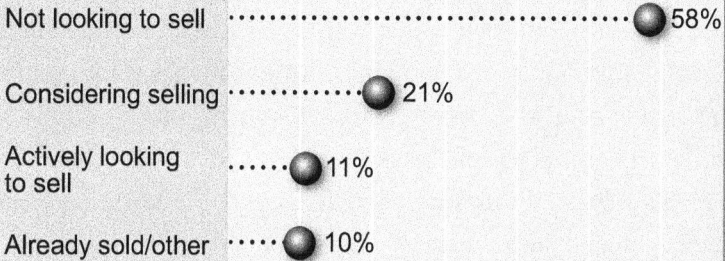

Not looking to sell	58%
Considering selling	21%
Actively looking to sell	11%
Already sold/other	10%

Source: Medical Economics, May 22, 2013.

Spencer said MAs are trained not to seem like they are encouraging appointments in order to avoid being viewed as marketers.

The second layer of patient engagement is PFP's patient portal. Patients have password-protected access to their medical records. They make appointments, request drug refills, pay bills or pose questions to providers. He does not charge for email access, and patients get answers within 24 hours. He has more patients on his portal than any other U.S. customer of his portal-creator vendor.

Once patients set appointments, they immediately get a text message and a reminder the night before that may include a message to fast. Texting has cut the no-show rate by 70 percent. Spencer also uses and monitors social media. His practice uses Twitter and Facebook to announce practice updates, flu-shot clinics and encouraging tweets.

Spencer embraces team care. Most of the PFP physicians can handle patient panels of 6,000 to 9,000 patients, because of liberal use of physician assistants and nurse practitioners. He said about 80 percent of primary care can be performed by mid-level clinicians. Patients are reassured that they have immediate access to a physician during an appointment if that is necessary.

Spencer said the live phone-answering and technology efforts were aimed at doing what was right for the patient. However, the increased staffing has more than paid for itself. He said the two biggest appointment generators were MAs talking to patients about whether they should come to the physician's office, and providers talking to patients about gaps in care or conditions that are not under control.

The micro practice

In 2004, Dr. Pamela Wible could not get out of bed. She was in a deep depression over her plight. She was living her life-long dream of being a family doctor—and she hated it. She had worked in a series of primary-care clinics, churning through as many as 30 patients a day.

After weeks of bed rest in 2004, she had an epiphany. She wanted to open her own clinic from scratch. She used a series of community meetings with local residents to ask them what they believed would be an ideal clinic. Ultimately, they wanted simple, affordable access. That's what Wible wanted as well.

In 2005, she opened her cozy office in the Tamarack Wellness Center in a residential section of south Eugene, Ore. The office complex includes an eclectic mix of therapies, including yoga, massage, counseling and a heated pool.

A significant proportion of those who attended Wible's

meetings became her patients. Wible could bike to work and set her own hours. She did everything: the billing, scheduling, answering the phone whenever possible.

Wible did not know it, but she was designing her office in the image of the Ideal Medical Practice (IMP). The model, often called a micro practice, was studied with the financial support of the Physicians Foundation in 2006. Drs. L. Gordon Moore and John Wasson found that IMP physicians were netting an average of $123,000 per year while seeing an average of 11 patients a day. The average IMP overhead was 35 percent of gross revenue, compared with 60 percent for a typical family practice. They found that nearly twice as many chronic-disease sufferers reported they were helped "a lot" by IMP physicians as at typical physician practices.

Wible said there are about eight IMPs in Eugene, including two others in the wellness center: Leigh Saint-Louis and Orestes Gutierrez, both of whom were influenced by Wible.

Wible had been practicing three afternoons a week, handling about 500 patients, but has cut back even that abbreviated schedule to promote her briskly selling autobiography, *Pet Goats & Pap Smears*. She is using the book proceeds to promote IMP.

Her 280-square-foot office has the feel of a living room. She has a basket of knickknacks, which she gives to patients if she is late for an appointment (which rarely happens) or as a reward for good health habits.

Her overhead is only about $10,000 a year—far below the IMP average—and she earns more than she did working for a group practice.

"I could rake it in next month if I wanted to," she said of her income. She prefers the light schedule instead.

She was able to get an 86 percent discount on her malpractice insurance because she works part time and took risk-reduction classes. About 80 percent of her patients have health insurance, which she bills through a free online clearinghouse. Most of her uninsured patients take advantage of her 40 percent discount for those who pay in advance. She refuses to take Medicare because of the administrative hassles.

She does her own scheduling and is readily available to patients by phone or email. She makes occasional house calls, and has had impromptu consultations with patients in grocery aisles and at the Department of Motor Vehicles office.

Wible is adamant about instilling patient self-reliance.

"Sometimes I think we infantilize patients," she said. "We've created monsters who are begging for refills. I handle it more like a peer relationship. They need fewer appointments, because I spend more time with them. They don't have anxiety about not having their questions answered."

Wible says she has encountered plenty of skepticism when evangelizing about IMP on the road:

"Doctors tell me, 'This would never work in Beverly Hills or Orange County or Dallas.' They say I live on 'Planet Oregon.' Doctors are not big risk takers. They don't like to stray far from the herd. But doctors need to be happy. If they aren't, that's a toxic environment for patients.

"I often hear, 'If everyone did this (IMP), we wouldn't have enough doctors.' I plan to practice until I'm 90, unless I become demented. There are retired doctors who are bored out of their minds. We could double the number of doctors. They're just not aware of this model."

Speaking with Wible's patients at her office one afternoon, a visitor finds them extolling her virtues. They talk about how she treats "the whole person."

One patient said she found Wible after having had a bad experience at a large practice.

"She's like an old-fashioned country doctor, or like Marcus Welby. I wouldn't go to another doctor if I was paid to do so. She gives me enough information to treat myself." This woman said she had recently encountered her former doctor, who had treated her for 30 years. "She didn't recognize me," the patient said. "She looked at me as if I somehow looked familiar."

Leigh Saint-Louis is one of two other micro practices at Tamarack.

Saint-Louis said her practice reflects the fact that she has the heart of a social worker.

"I have a very noisy conscience. I want to take care of the sick, poor and medically complex. I take care of patients who don't have anyone else to take care of them," she said.

She entered medical school after spending most of her 20s raising her children and working as a community organizer, lay health advocate and perinatal educator.

Saint-Louis had earned an undergraduate degree in biochemistry from the University of Illinois, and spent her residency at an inner-city hospital in Milwaukee. She was not interested in joining what she calls "the medical establishment." She ran across an article written by Moore on IMP and was smitten.

She was attracted to Eugene's bohemian culture, although she quickly discovered that the community was hostile to Western medicine.

She said residents tell her, "I hate doctors. I won't go to see one and I won't take medicine."

She has built her practice mostly through word of mouth. Word spread quickly that she treats the uninsured.

Saint-Louis has a flat rate for each visit: $60, due upon arrival. She decided on that amount after she did a Facebook survey, asking people what they thought would be fair. Most said $50 to $100. She initially took insurance reimbursement when she opened her practice in 2009, but got rid of it once it was feasible to do so. She said she has a long-standing hostility toward insurance companies, having been denied coverage herself because of a pre-existing condition. She barters her primary care needs with another physician.

Saint-Louis works 20 hours a week, has overhead of about $1,000 a month and earns about $50,000 a year. She said that is about one-third of what other IMP physicians make, and she is fine with that. Her income, she said, is about equal to that of a math teacher, which she believes is fair—especially since she is working part time.

"Doctors don't have to be afraid" of becoming an IMP, she said. "The only barrier is your own preconceptions. You're the boss. If you don't want to go into the office (on days without appointments), you're not letting anyone down. If you don't get paperwork done, the only one who cares is you."

Saint-Louis keeps in contact with other IMP physicians through a listserv. She said most of her colleagues are "refugees from large group practices. Universally, they say they would never go back."

Orestes Gutierrez, the third IMP physician at Tamarack, had had it. He was unhappy practicing at a large clinic. He perpetually was an hour behind because he insisted on spending more time with his patients. When his contract was about to expire, he began looking around. Leigh Saint-Louis was his family physician, so he was intrigued by IMPs. He interviewed with a smaller practice that offered him the opportunity to see only 10 patients a day and keep 45 percent of the reimbursement he generated.

His wife, a medical school dropout, offered to be his business manager if he started an IMP.

"We're going to take 100 percent (of the reimbursement)," she told him.

In only his third month, Gutierrez pulled in more than $18,000 of gross revenue. His monthly overhead was $1,100. He worked four days a week and saw fewer than five patients a day that month. He plans to cap his practice at no more than 10 patient visits a day.

Unlike Saint-Louis, he is in-network with most major insurers and said about 40 percent of his business is Medicare Advantage.

Gutierrez spends about an hour with new patients and for physicals, and 30 minutes for return visits. He gets about a half-dozen emails a day, which he dispatches quickly because they generally are simple questions. If the conversations become involved, he insists patients come in for a visit. Although his patients have complete access to him, his phone rarely rings after 5 p.m. He uses eFax for prescriptions, and his electronic medical records system is free.

"In my old practice," he said, "we used triage nurses and office employees to do what I do in two seconds. That is the administrative burden of medicine. Here when you order a prescription refill, it is approved by me. That's a much safer way to practice. I have my finger on every single aspect of the practice. Any doctor can go completely solo. It's simple. You can do it if you can hit 'enter' and 'return' on the keyboard. But you have to be comfortable with people. Some doctors prefer to spend five minutes with the patient and say 'Do this.' You can't be afraid to get deeply connected with patients. You have to have the right personality."

Gutierrez concedes he would have a difficult time taking on the workload without his wife's help.

"I could do this full time if I didn't have a wife and kids," he added.

Concierge medicine

Dr. Cyrus Peikari sees no more than 200 patients. After nearly a decade of physician leadership positions at two Dallas hospitals, he opened an IMP in 2005 and transformed it into a concierge medical practice in 2010.

Concierge medicine is also called retainer-based medicine or boutique medicine. Physicians typically charge patients a monthly or annual fee. Concierge doctors limit the number of patients they see and offer enhanced access, longer appointments and highly customized patient care. Many, including Peikari, do not take insurance.

Two kinds of patients tend to be attracted to retainer-based practices: high-income patients who place great value on their time and on ready access, and patients with complex medical conditions.

It is a model designed to promote doctor-patient relationships, increase face-to-face time, reduce physician workload, instill in patients a sense of personal responsibility for their health and combat administrative waste.

Peikari points out that the typical physician office has 4.5 employees for every doctor. Because he is cash only and does not accept insurance, his office consists of himself and a medical assistant.

He encourages his patients to have insurance for catastrophic medical events.

Cost can be a significant barrier for patients who want concierge care. Peikari's fee is $360 a month, which he acknowledges places him among the higher-priced retainer practices. He said he based his rate on the $12 an average person spends on "junk food" each day. He believes he can show a return on the patients' investment by saving them hundreds of dollars monthly, weaning them off medications and helping forestall chronic conditions by coaching them on proper health behaviors.

"The idea is to spend it on health care and get more for your investment. The reason people pay for concierge medicine is that they see results. They need someone to believe in them," he said.

Many U.S. physicians would like to take the leap into concierge medicine. About 16 percent of U.S. physicians said they planned to switch to a cash-only practice within three years, according to a survey by physician recruitment firm Merritt Hawkins. A 2011 Deloitte Center for Health Solutions survey asked physicians what they considered an ideal practice setting. The top two answers were: an administrative role in a large health organization, or a concierge medical practice.

"Everyone (in health care) is in transition," Peikari said. "The market is eliminating traditional practices, which are going bankrupt. It is becoming either concierge medicine or mass medicine. Any doctor can do this."

Dr. Paul Cary also is a Dallas concierge physician. But while Peikari would be considered a "pure" concierge doctor, Cary is more of a hybrid model. His patients pay $1,500 for an extensive annual physical, but pay no monthly fee—and the doctor accepts insurance.

Cary is part of the MDVIP network of concierge physicians. The 600-physician network, owned by Procter & Gamble, operates in 41 states and treats more than 200,000 patients. MDVIP physicians remain independent, but they pay a franchise fee per patient for marketing support and other services.

Cary previously had a 2,000-patient panel. From that, he was able to create his current patient base of 350. About 30 percent of his previous practice consisted of Medicare patients. Now it is about 60 percent. He said his patients are in their 40s, 50s and 60s, value extensive preventive care or have multiple medical problems.

Cary said the conversion "is definitely worthwhile. If (doctors) can do it, they are going to be glad they did. Insurance companies have been squeezing physicians more and more, and you have to see more patients. When I started 25 years ago, internists saw 12-15 patients a day. Now it's 25 a day."

As a concierge physician, he sees four to 12 patients a day.

The independent practice association

An independent practice association (IPA) is a contractual organization of independent physicians that can be a single or multi-specialty group. Physicians maintain their independence, but as part of the IPA they are able to negotiate collectively with payers on issues other than reimbursement rates.

Managed-care plans, health systems or accountable care organizations (ACOs) can contract with an IPA, which in turn contracts with independent physicians to provide services. However, antitrust laws do not allow IPAs to negotiate as a group with commercial insurance companies for higher rates.

IPAs also can help physicians improve their operations. They can provide case management and data analysis, supply back-office services or serve as a purchasing organization to garner discounts on supplies and equipment. An IPA allows physicians to spread the cost of typical practice expenses and reduce the administrative burden. IPAs also have emerged as a tool to allow small physician practices to participate in value-based medicine.

IPAs were initially formed in the 1990s to facilitate capitation rates with managed-care organizations. Some IPAs vanished because they negotiated inadequate rates to cover practice expenses. However, many survived and thrived. The IPA Association of America claims 677 members, composed of 303,000 physicians in 39 states.

Dave Gans, vice president of innovation and research for MGMA, told *Repertoire* magazine in 2011, "In my opinion, we'll see a resurgence of the IPA. It provides the opportunity for contract and negotiating clout; it also offers the ability to sustain information systems on behalf of many of its doctors and to help the communication function. Doctors need electronic health records, but they oftentimes need that bridge (that the IPA can afford). The IPA becomes the alternative option for the doctor to remain independent."

IPAs are organized ideally to become physician-run ACOs themselves.

Dr. Wayne Pan, chief medical officer of Individual Practice

Association Medical Group of Santa Clara County, Calif., told *Physicians Practice*: "For many years, in fact, IPAs have been aligning physicians to achieve a wide variety of goals—including managed-care-style models for reducing costs and increasing quality of care. Compared to many hospital-led ACO initiatives, therefore, practice associations have an advantage— hospitals may have to build from the ground up when coordinating diverse groups of physicians and specialists in the community, while provider groups often already have the structure in place, including arrangements with regional hospitals and health networks. In addition, many IPAs have had extensive experience working within risk-bearing arrangements for some time now, making them ripe for ACO development which incorporates similar shared savings concepts."

Dr. Steven Davis, medical director of Torrance, Calif.-based HealthCare Partners IPA, said: "Besides all the structure, tools and support, the IPA brings the strength of size and critical mass that allows the small practice to participate in larger group arenas such as ACOs. Beyond their clinical-care management, they provide the contracting, analytics and business logistics to build, qualify and sustain an ACO. This complete clinical and business picture is not readily available to most small practices or even some other forms of health-care organizations that will try to form ACOs."

Cary, the concierge physician, is treasurer of the 1,400-physician Genesis Physician Group and has been a member for 15 years. Although the IPA cannot directly negotiate prices on commercial payer contracts, it does vet the contracts on non-financial issues. During a recent contract discussion, for example, it requested more than 80 changes and received more than half of its requests. Cary said Genesis also can encourage payers to offer contracts that are more generous and attract pay-for-performance programs. Doctors such as Cary also benefit from IPA group purchasing and credentialing services.

Dr. Jim Walton, chief executive officer of Genesis, said, "IPAs are growing because doctors are choosing to stay independent. They always wanted to be entrepreneurs."

Clinical integration

Clinical integration (CI) is a specific legal arrangement that allows physicians and hospitals to collaborate on improving efficiency and quality while remaining independent of each other. Physicians generally agree to improve performance, serve on committees and change their practices to accommodate integration. Physicians sign an agreement to practice evidence-based medicine as defined by their peers, to share their clinical data, and to use standardized clinical protocols. Although hospitals typically organize the networks, they generally are led and operated by physicians.

CI enjoys a safe harbor from antitrust rules. In 1996 the Federal Trade Commission (FTC) and Department of Justice jointly offered this opportunity to negotiate rates and quality bonuses collectively with commercial payers. The FTC has issued four advisory opinions since then, three of which have been positive. The networks that have gotten the FTC's blessing had several key features, including clinical guidelines and protocols, digital measurement of quality measures, ongoing process-improvement mechanisms and willingness to share data with payers.

This legal safety zone is a powerful advantage. However, CI efforts also brand practices in a positive way, signaling to patients and payers that they are committed to delivering consistent clinical quality.

As of late 2012, there were more than 500 U.S. CI organizations, which barely existed a few years ago.

A prime example of CI is Advocate Health Care. Advocate was named one of the nation's top health systems based on clinical performance in 2011 by Thomson Reuters. Advocate is the largest health system in Illinois and one of the largest healthcare providers in the Midwest, operating more than 250 sites of care. Among its facilities are 12 hospitals with more than 3,300 beds, Chicago's largest medical group, with more than 200 locations.

Its CI program, called Advocate Physician Partners (APP), includes more than 1,100 primary-care physicians and 2,700 specialists. Of those, 2,900 are independent solo or small group practices, with the balance being employed by Advocate.

APP focuses measuring and monitoring on five broad categories: enhancing clinical outcomes, improving patient safety, adopting clinical technology, improving patient satisfaction and increasing efficiency.

Physicians receive quarterly "report cards" upon which bonuses are determined. Advocate publishes an annual "Value Report" on CI measures. APP contracts with every major Chicago-area health plan.

The program started in 2004, with 36 measures directed largely at primary-care physicians. It has grown to include nearly 160 measures of clinical effectiveness, efficiency, patient safety and patient experience.

According to Dr. Lee Sacks, Advocate Health chief medical officer, CI may address three overarching challenges for delivery reform: the limitations of fee-for-service reimbursement; the need for infrastructure for small practices to improve outcomes and prove quality, and barriers to optimal physician-hospital collaboration.

Advocate has invested about $100 million in IT infrastructure to nurture the network. APP has 70 outpatient-care navigators who work with its primary-care physicians to address the needs of its sickest 3 to 5 percent of patients.

APP was able to distribute $38 million in incentive funds to its physicians in 2009, up from $25 million in 2007, because of clinical improvements.

Advocate and Blue Cross Blue Shield of Illinois launched an ACO in 2010 called AdvocateCare, covering about 250,000 PPO and 125,000 HMO members. In its first year, it was able to decrease inpatient days by more than 12 percent.

In 2012, Advocate became a participant in the Centers for Medicare & Medicaid Services (CMS) Medicare Shared Savings Program, providing care to about 120,000 Medicare fee-for-service beneficiaries.

Many consider CI an evolutionary step toward ACO creation. Although ACOs and CI efforts share some similar characteristics, there are key differences, according to consultant Kaufman Hall. ACOs are designed to meet quality and cost-efficiency goals primarily in one legal entity, while CI is geared toward integrating hospital, primary care and specialty care. ACOs generally assume financial risk for their patients while CI programs generally do not include risk-based shared-savings incentives.

According to the American Hospital Association, hospital CI efforts cover a broad spectrum. At one end, a targeted effort would include a hospital and a small subset of its voluntary medical staff to address a specific procedure or condition. At the other end of the spectrum, a health system's wholly owned hospitals and physician groups are integrated financially.

Advocate's PHO would be considered somewhere in the middle of that continuum, because it weaves together employed and independent physicians across a broad spectrum of initiatives and includes negotiations with health plans.

Prashant Deshpande, a pediatrician at Southwest Pediatrics in suburban Chicago, has participated in APP almost since it began in the mid-1990s. He said he appreciates the hybrid model of remaining independent while being able to benefit from group purchasing, clinical benchmarking and APP's ability to craft favorable insurance contracts.

"I want to do things the way I want to. My office can reach me day and night. I take pride in that. If I was employed, I would lose autonomy, independence and the pride of being in private practice," he said.

William Hulesch, a family physician in Downers Grove, Ill., has been with APP since it began. He said the main advantage of CI is the ability to identify specialists and share patient information quickly and seamlessly. He also likes the ability to prove quality of patient care and be compensated for that.

"When you divide it (the incentive money) by 12 months and five practitioners, it is not a lot of money. But the system incentivizes you to give good medical care and actually get paid for it," he said.

Carrie Nelson, APP medical director, said insurers tend to use their own quality measures when negotiating contracts. However, APP is able to get payers to agree to a common set of measures, which allows APP to build a common infrastructure around those measures.

Nelson recommends that physicians looking to join CI efforts verify that there is strong physician leadership and transparency about bonus payments. She said she has seen PHOs that do not share bonus money with participating physicians.

Consultant Kaufman Hall offers the following advice for those wanting to create a CI program:

- Physician leadership is required for both CI and ACOs.
- CI incremental change is achievable regardless of its size.
- Technology is the largest investment for CI programs and ACOs.
- The physician network and clinical measures should be developed gradually.
- Planning is critical to success.
- Antitrust issues should be considered as CI programs move toward ACOs.

Returning to private practice

New York orthopedic physician Louis McIntyre is one of the relatively few who returned to independent practice after being employed by a hospital following the sale of Westchester Orthopedic Associates (see page 115). He left White Plains Hospital after his initial contract expired. Although he had to forgo three months of accounts receivable, he was able to reconstitute much of his desired cash flow within a few months.

McIntyre said he suspects—without having hard data—that the second contracts offered to employed physicians are far less lucrative than the initial ones. He recounted the experience of physicians who sold their Westchester County practice to a

Connecticut hospital and ran into a brick wall when renegotiating employment contracts.

"The hospital administrator said, 'We own you. There is nothing you can do.' Bottom line, these guys just played hardball. They treat doctors like commodities. Once that happens, your salary is at risk." McIntyre said.

McIntyre recommends that physicians seek to become joint-venture partners with hospitals rather than become employees. Doing so allows physicians to maintain their practice autonomy, charge the hospital's negotiated insurance rates and create ancillary revenue opportunities.

If physicians do sell their practices and become hospital employees, McIntyre suggests they hire a health-care attorney to help negotiate as much autonomy as possible and minimize restrictive covenants in case they decide not to renew their contracts. If departing employment and seeking to regain independent practice, the physician can use leverage by saying he or she will continue to use the hospital "so they are nice to you," he said.

McIntyre said it may be difficult for some who would like to hang out their shingle after having been employed. Young, employed physicians who have never established a practice would have a hard time without an established patient base. Going without income for several months is difficult. Physicians who say they only want to practice medicine are not good candidates for independence.

"If that's all you want to do, be a hospital employee and don't complain. You have to be good at billing and collections. You have to bite the bullet," he said.

Physician leadership

Dr. Robert Monteiro, a New Bern, N.C., internist, was part of a practice that was sold to CarolinaEast Medical Center. He signed a three-year contract in January 2011.

At first, the transition was seamless. He saw the same patients and worked the same schedule. He enjoyed the economic security of a large, successful organization. He liked the fact that he was paid based on Relative Value Units.

Then things started to change. Monteiro said CarolinaEast decided to consolidate equipment. Patients now had to go elsewhere for blood work, mammograms and bone-density tests. He said the system then clinically integrated EMR "in a way that would not have been done if the organization was physician-run."

Then his practice schedule changed. That was enough for Monteiro. He planned to complete his contract and join a physician-led clinic associated with the University of North Carolina in January 2014.

"It's different practicing as an employee vs. being an owner. My experience has shown me that it is crucial that doctors be involved in administration as well as the delivery of care. Without that input, doctors and patients both suffer," he said.

Physician leadership is not necessarily the path to physician independence, but it can be the next best thing for working conditions.

Most patients would be surprised by how little involvement their physicians have in running health-care organizations.

The vast majority of U.S. hospitals are led by non-physicians. It was not always that way. A century ago, about one out of three hospitals were led by physicians. That has dwindled to less than 2 percent of hospitals.

According to a HealthLeaders survey, more than one-third of hospital and health-system CEOs said they had no physicians on their senior leadership teams, which includes titles of senior vice president and higher. About half said 1 to 20 percent of their senior leadership teams were composed of physicians.

There is a movement afoot to put physicians into leadership positions, because delivery reform law is changing the health-care landscape. Health-care organizations now must focus as much on quality as financial performance. Patients and policymakers are demanding greater transparency, patient safety, cost-effectiveness and accountability.

For all this to happen, physicians need a strong voice.

The American College of Physician Executives said it taught physician leadership courses for about 200 days in 2011, which is double the average of previous years.

The need for physician leadership has trickled down to medical schools. The combined enrollment in M.D./Ph.D., M.D./J.D. and M.D./MBA programs has increased by more than a third from 2002 to 2011, according to the Association of American Medical Colleges. The vast majority are enrolled in M.D./Ph.D. programs.

Business training for physicians has been growing steadily. More than 50 percent of medical schools now offer a joint M.D./MBA degree, according to Dr. Maria Chandler, head of University of California at Irvine's Medical School and president of the Association of MD MBA Programs. Physicians make up about half of the enrollees in the school's health-care executive MBA program.

About seven out of 10 physicians say an administrative role

in a large health-care delivery system would be an ideal occupational setting despite the pressure, according to a Deloitte Center for Health Solutions survey.

A 2011 study by a British researcher found that hospital quality scores were about 25 percent higher at hospitals led by physicians. Scores for cancer care were even higher at physician-led hospitals. The same researcher conducted a similar study on National Basketball Association coaches, which found that teams coached by former star players improved substantially during the first 12 months of their being hired.

Like star athletes, physician leaders can be role models for the medical staff and clearly have an advantage when recruiting clinical talent. They have instant credibility because they have "walked the walk" as a healer.

Traditional physician training emphasizes individual performance and evaluation. Doctors are taught to be autonomous thinkers. As medical residents, they spend long apprenticeships as subordinates, usually under command-and-control mentors. They are trained for individual contribution. Collaboration and teamwork are foreign concepts.

Physicians by nature are fiercely independent. Doctors are highly trained scientists used to having the final say on how they treat their patients. Many see the study of leadership as weak and lacking the rigor of science.

Dr. Jim Jacobson, an Arlington, Texas, physician and consultant for large medical groups and insurance companies, said, "Physicians have a unique position in the health-care arena. They are at the center of patient care. They can look at patient care from the inside out. If they are a physician leader, they can also look at it from the outside in, taking into account both the clinical and business aspects of the organization."

Some health-care executives simply believe physicians cannot lead. Jacobson said a hospital association executive spoke to a graduate course he was teaching and joked that "physician leadership" was an oxymoron.

Physician leadership is broader than simply running hospitals. Doctors also serve as chief medical officers, head clinical departments and often serve on hospital boards of directors. However, they too often are promoted because of clinical or academic success rather than leadership skill or readiness.

Dr. Carl Couch, president of the Baylor Health Care System's ACO in Dallas, said, "Doctors are a highly educated group of people. But their education and career is mostly technical and clinical. The whole subject of physician leadership training has only received attention in the last 10-15 years."

Dr. Russell Dickey, former chief of staff at USMD Hospital in Arlington, Texas, said USMD identifies four to six promising candidates each year for weekend training geared to cultivate physician leaders. A physician working in a hospital, he said, cannot "just show up for work anymore. You have to participate. There is a lot of work behind the scenes for the hospital to be successful. The hospital requires physicians be much more involved than they used to be. And that's a good thing."

Most hospital-based physicians agree. According to a survey by consultant PwC, more than nine out of 10 such physicians believe they should be more involved in hospital executive leadership and management.

Physician leaders can take patient care and advocacy to a higher level, transforming their professional ethics and compassion into institutional policies and affecting far more lives.

Evidence indicates that physicians who serve as chief executive officers have higher job satisfaction than those who spend their careers treating individual patients.

Physician leaders have a natural empathy for, and credibility with, front-line physicians who are practicing in an increasingly demanding environment.

To keep clinical skills fresh, many physician leaders continue to see patients. According to a survey of chief medical officers at health systems and hospitals, about 15 percent continued clinical duties despite heavy administrative responsibilities. A separate survey found that more than two out of three physician executives continue to practice medicine, with nearly half saying it is a job requirement.

Joel Shalowitz, director of the health-industry management program at Northwestern University's Kellogg School of Management in Chicago, said, "Doctors don't understand the language of management. That breeds distrust. Health-care managers have made it their business to understand the language of medicine, but the opposite is not true. Leadership training helps develop a common language."

McIntyre, the New York orthopedic physician who left hospital employment, is blunt about the disadvantages of non-physician leadership.

He said hospital administrators "have no idea what they're doing" when tasked with running a physician practice.

"Hospital administrators have no clue about patient care," he said. "They just want to make sure all the i's are dotted and T's are crossed. They'll bend doctors into pretzels to make sure they are meeting regulations even if what they're doing makes no sense. They are completely clueless, almost disturbingly so."

References

CHAPTER 1

"Dr. Don McCanne..." McCanne D. How would Marcus Welby, M.D., fare in an ACO? pnhp.org/blog/2011/04/26/how-would-marcus-welby-m-d-fare-in-an-aco/. April 26, 2011. Accessed July 8, 2013.

"Nearly half..." Personal health care expenditures, by source of funds and type of expenditure: United States, selected years 1960-2010.

"In a 2005 survey..." Physician salary, compensation and practice surveys. Merritt Hawkins. merritthawkins.com/compensation-surveys.aspx. Accessed July 8, 2013.

"Physician recruiter Merritt Hawkins CEO..." Testimony of Mark Smith, President, Merritt Hawkins before the U.S. House Committee on Small Business. smallbusiness.house.gov/uploadedfiles/7-19_smith_testimony.pdf. July 19, 2012. Accessed October 9, 2012.

"In 1973..." Hadley J Cancer JC, Willke RJ, Feder J, Cohen AB. Young physicians most and least likely to have second thoughts about a career in medicine. *Acad Med.* 1992;67:180-190.

"Darrell Kirch..." Tanner L. Forget Marcus Welby: Today's docs want a real life. Associated Press. September 2, 2012.

"New Hampshire..." Wortmann RL. From "Marcus Welby" to "Scrubs." *Clinical Psychiatry News.* Vol. 37, No. 9. September 2009.

"In November 2012..." Statement by CPR purchases on price and quality transparency in health care. Catalyst for Payment Reform. catalyzepaymentreform.org/uploads/Price_Transparency_Statement.pdf Accessed November 18, 2012.

"Billionaire investor Warren Buffet..." Lazarus D. Warren Buffett calls health care the 'tapeworm' of U.S. economy. *The Los Angeles Times.* July 13, 2012.

"Many other nations..." Levey NNH. Is world outpacing U.S. on health care? The Los Angeles Times. May 14, 2012.

"However, the Institute of Medicine..." Institute of Medicine. The healthcare imperative: Lowering costs and improving outcomes. Workshop series summary. Washington, D.C.: National Academies Press, 2010.

"Physician Harvey Fineberg, IOM president..." Fineberg HV. A successful and sustainable health system—how to get there from here. *N Engl J Med.* 2012;366(11):1020-1027.

"Bruce Vladeck..." Vladeck BC. Managed care's fifteen minutes of fame. *J Health Polit Polic.* 1999;24:1207-1211.

"Robert Berenson and colleagues..." Berenson RA, Hammons T, Gans D et al. A house is not a home: Keeping patients at the center of practice redesign. *Health Aff.* 2008;27(5):1219-1230.

"Yale Professor Emeritus..." Marmor T, Oberlander J. From HMOs to ACOs: The quest for the Holy Grail in U.S. health policy. *J Gen Intern Med.* 2012;27(9):1215-1218.

"As a rule of thumb..." Fuchs VR. Major trends in the U.S. health economy since 1950. *N Engl J Med.* 2012;366(11):973-977.

"Despite this..." Auerbach DL, Kellermann AL. A decade of health care cost grow has wiped out real income gains for an average U.S. family. *Health Aff.* 2011;30(9):1630-1636.

"Primary-care physicians' share..." Berenson, op cit.

"If payers cut reimbursement..." Aaron HJ, Ginsburg PB. Is health spending excessive? If so, what can we do about it. *Health Aff.* 2008;28(5):1260-1275.

"However, doctors control 80 cents..." Health reform and the decline of physician private practice. The Physicians Foundation website. physiciansfoundation.org/uploadedFiles/Health%20Reform%20and%20the%20 Decline%20of%20Physician%20Private%20Practice.pdf. October 2010. Accessed May 11, 2011.

"In its 2012 survey..." Newport F. Congress retains low honesty rating. gallup.com/poll/159035/congress-retains-low-honesty-rating.aspx. December 3, 2012. Accessed December 4, 2012.

"More than 3 out of 4..." Sanger-Katz M. Why we trust doctors. *National Journal.* nationaljournal.com/features/restoration-calls/why-we-trust-doctors-20120419?page=1. April 26, 2012. Accessed December 4, 2012.

"About 4 out of 10..." Elliott VS. 41% of Americans voice confidence in health care system. *American Medical News.* July 12, 2012.

"Stanford University professors..." Fuchs VR, Milstein A. The $640 billion question—Why does cost-effective care diffuse so slowly? *N Engl J Med.* 2011;364(21):1985-1987.

"Only 15 percent..." Schoen C, Osborn R, Squires D, et al. A survey of primary care doctors in ten countries shows progress in use of health information technology, less in other areas. *Health Aff.* 2012;31(12)2805-2816.

"According to a large study..." Shanafelt TD, Boone S, Tan L, et al. Burnout and satisfaction with work-life balance among U.S. physicians relative to the general U.S. population. *Arch Intern Med.* 2012;172(18):1377-1385.

"A separate survey..." Physician Wellness Services and Cejka search physician stress and burnout survey. physicianwellnessservices.com/news/stresssurvey.php. Accessed December 10, 2012.

"Physicians have the highest suicide rate..." Noonan D. Doctors who kill themselves. Newsweek. thedailybeast.com/newsweek/2008/04/19/doctors-who-kill-themselves.html April 19, 2008. Accessed December 4, 2012; Gold KJ, Sen A, Schwenk TL. Details on suicide among U.S. physicians: Data from the National Violent Death Reporting System. *Gen Hosp Psychiatry.* sciencedirect.com/science/article/pii/S016383431200268X November 2, 2012. Accessed December 4, 2012.

"A study of surgeons..." Dyrbye LN, Freischlag J, Kaups KI, et al. Work-home conflicts have a substantial impact on career decisions that affect the adequacy of the surgical workforce. Arch Surg. 2012;147(10):933-939.

"Nearly half..." Dyrbye LN, Thomas MR, Massie FS, et al. Burn-out and suicidal ideation among U.S. medical students. Ann Intern Med. 2008;149(5):334-341.

"It is troubling..." The Physicians Foundation. Practice arrangements among young physicians and their views regarding the future of the U.S. health care system. physiciansfoundation.org/uploads/default/Next_Generation_Physician_Survey.pdf. April 2012. Accessed December 4, 2012.

"Those physicians..." A sense of call and primary care physicians' satisfaction in treating smoking, alcoholism and obesity. Rasinski KA, Lawrence RE, Yoon JD, Curtin FA. Arch Intern Med. 2012;172(18):1423-1424; Del Canale S, Louis DZ, Maio V, et al. The relationship between physician empathy and disease complications: An empirical study of primary care physicians and their diabetic patients in Parma, Italy. *Acad Med.* 2012;87:1243-1249.

"A survey of hospital..." 2013 survey of alumni satisfaction & health system trends. Merritt Hawkins. 2013. trinity.edu/Documents/Health%20Care%20Admin/Trinity_Health_Care_Survey.pdf. Accessed November 1, 2013.

"According to a survey..." Nurse practitioners may have higher job satisfaction than physicians, survey says. *Medical Economics.* October 7, 2013.

CHAPTER 2

"Spending on physician..." Hartman M, Martin AB, Benson J, et al. National health spending in 2011: Overall growth remains low, but some payers and services show signs of acceleration. Health Aff. 2013;32(87-99.

"Three major studies..." Cutler DM, Sahni. If slow rate of health care spending growth persists, projections may be off by $770 billion. *Health Aff.* 2013;32(5):841-850; Assessing the effects of the economy on the recent slowdown in health spending. Kaiser Family Foundation. kff.org/health-costs/

issue-brief/assessing-the-effects-of-the-economy-on-the-recent-slowdown-in-health-spending-2/. April 22, 2013. Accessed June 6, 2013; Ryu AJ, Gibson TB, McKellar MR, Chernew ME. The slowdown in health care spending in 2009-11 reflected factors other than the weak economy and thus may persist. *Health Aff.* 2013;32(5):835-840; Lowrey A. Slowdown in health costs' rise may last as economy revives. *The New York Times.* May 6, 2013.

"By 2022..." Cuckler GA, Sisko AM, Keehan SP, et al. National health expenditure projections, 2012-22: Slow growth until coverage expands and economy improves. *Health Aff.* 2013; 32(10):1820-1831.

"However, Dartmouth researchers..." Fisher E, Goodman D, Skinner J, Bronner K. Health care spending, quality, and outcomes; more isn't always better," *A Dartmouth Atlas Project Topic Brief.* February 2009.

"According to Health Care Cost Institute..." Health Care Cost and Utilization Report: 2011. healthcostinstitute.org/2011report. September 2012. Accessed May 7, 2013.

"The ratio..." Ginsburg P. Reforming provider payment — the price side of the equation. *N Engl J Med.* 2011;365(1268-1270).

"A 2013 *Health Services Research*..." White C, Wu VY. How do hsopitals cope with sustained slow growth in Medicare prices. HSR. 2013; hschange.org/CONTENT/1385/1385.pdf. Accessed October 30, 2013.

"Research shows..." White C. Contrary to cost-shift theory, lower Medicare hospital payment rates for inpatient care lead to lower private rates. Health Aff. 2013;32(5):935-943; He D, Mellor JM. Hospital volume responses to Medicare's outpatient prospective payment system: Evidence from Florida. *Journal of Health Economics.* 2012;31(5):730-743.

"Census data bear out..." O'Hara B, Caswell K. Health status, health insurance, and medical services utilization: 2010. census.gov/prod/2012pubs/p70-133.pdf. October 2012. Accessed October 7, 2012.

"However, physician visits..." Cook B. As more patients see physicians again, health plan earnings drop. *American Medical News.* September 3, 2012.

"Even so ..." The use of medicines in the United States: Review of 2011. IMS Institute for Healthcare Informatics. imshealth.com/ims/Global/Content/Insights/IMS%20Institute%20for%20Healthcare%20Informatics/IHII_Medicines_in_U.S_Report_2011.pdf. April 4, 2012. Accessed October 8, 2012.

"A Stanford University analysis..." Claxton G, Levitt L. The economy and medical care. The Henry J. Kaiser Family Foundation Health Reform Source. healthreform.kff.org/notes-on-health-insurance-and-reform/2011/november/the-economy-and-medical-care.aspx. November 15, 2011. Accessed February 2, 2012.

"More than 9 million people..." Cawley J. Moriya AS, Simon KI. The impact of the macroeconomy on health insurance coverage: Evidence from the Great Recession. NBER Working Paper No. 17600. nber.org/papers/ w17600. November 2011. Accessed February 3, 2012.

"Fewer than half..." Driscoll AK, Bernstein AB. Health and access to care among employed and unemployed adults: United States, 2009–2010. NCHS Data Brief, no 83. Hyattsville, MD: National Center for Health Statistics. January 2012.

"Employees with high-deductible..." Galbraith AA, Soumerai SB, Ross-Degnan D, Rosenthan MB, Gay C, Lieu TA. Delayed and forgone care for families with chronic conditions in high-deductible health plans. *J Gen Intern Med.* ncbi.nlm.nih.gov/pubmed/22249829. January 18, 2012. Accessed February 2, 2012.

"The share of employees..." Employer health benefits 2011 annual survey. Kaiser Family Foundation. ehbs.kff.org/. September 27, 2011. Accessed February 2, 2012.

"Researchers point to..." Holahan J, Blumberg L, McMurrow S, Zuckerman S, Waidmann T, Stockley K. Containing the growth of spending in the U.S. health system. Urban Institute. urban.org/uploadedpdf/412419-Containing-the-Growth-of-Spending-in-the-US-Health-System.pdf. October 2011. Accessed October 8, 2012.

"Employers held..." Employers held health benefit cost growth to 4.1 percent in 2012, the smallest in 15 years. mercer.com/press-releases/1491670November 14, 2012. Accessed December 5, 2012.

"Experts say..." Lowrey A. In hopeful sign, health spending is flattening out. *The New York Times.* April 28, 2012.

"According to..." Health care budget deficit calculator. Center for Economic and Policy Research. cepr.net/calculators/hc/hc-calculator.html. Accessed October 7, 2012.

"During the recession..." Bradford JW, Knott DG, Levine EH, Zemmel RS. Accounting for the cost of U.S. health care. McKinsey Center for U.S. Health System Reform. healthreform.mckinsey.com/Home/Insights/Latest_thinking/Accounting_for_the_cost_of_US_health_care.aspx. December 2011. Accessed February 2, 2012.

"Health costs reached another..." Consumer price index – April 2011. U.S. Bureau of Labor Statistics website. bls.gov/news.release/archives/ cpi_08132010.pdf. August 13, 2010. Accessed May 24, 2011.

"Still, health spending is rising faster..." Health care spending in the United States and selected OECD countries, April 2011. Kaiser Family Foundation website. kff.org/insurance/snapshot/OECD042111.cfm. April 2011.

Accessed May 24, 2011.

"Health-care spending has slowed..." Kelland K. Growth in health spending grinding to a halt: OECD. in.reuters.com/article/2012/06/28/us-spending-oecd-idINBRE85R0PJ20120628. June 28, 2012. Accessed October 7, 2012.

"Peter Orszag, then-director..." Congressional testimony, Committee on the Budget, U.S. Senate. June 21, 2007.

"Federal health-care spending..." The budget and economic outlook: Fiscal years 2012 and 2022. Congressional Budget Office. cbo.gov/doc.cfm?index=12699. January 2012. Accessed February 3, 2012.

"The current trend..." Dentzer S. Rolling the rock up the mountain. *Health Aff.* 2009;28(5):1250-1252.

"Former Federal Reserve Chairman..." Irwin N, Montgomery L. Federal Reserve Chairman Ben Bernanke sounds a warning on growing deficit. *The Washington Post.* April 8, 2010.

"Americans clearly do not..." Murray M. NBC/WSJ poll: Voters deficit-worried but wary of cuts. msnbc.msn.com/id/41876558/ns/politics/. March 2, 2011. Accessed May 24, 2011; McClatchy-Marist poll. maristpoll.marist.edu/418-mcclatchy-marist-poll/ April 18, 2011. Accessed June 6, 2011.

"About half believe neither program..." AP-GfK poll: Medicare doesn't have to be cut. abcnews.go.com/Politics/wireStory?id=13662567. May 23, 2011. Accessed May 24, 2011.

"From late 2007 to February 2011..." Health sector economic indicators. Altarum Institute website. altarum.org/files/imce/CSHS-Labor-Brief_May%202011_051711.pdf. May 17, 2011. Accessed May 24, 2011.

"More than 41,000..." Planned layoffs total 40,289 in September. Challenger, Gray & Christmas. challengergray.com/press/PressRelease.aspx?PressUid=290. October 9, 2013. Accessed October 30, 2013.

"The average physician..." Casalino LP, Nicholson S, Gans DN, et al. What does it cost physician practices to interact with health insurance plans? *Health Aff.* 2009;28(4):w533-w543.

"According to CMS actuaries..." Shatto JD, Clemens MK. Office of the Actuarycms.gov/Research-Statistics-Data-and-Systems/Statistics-Trends-and-Reports/ReportsTrustFunds/Downloads/2013TRAlternativeScenario.pdf. May 31, 2013. Accessed October 14, 2013.

"The price tag..." The budget and economic outlook: Fiscal years 2013 to 2023. Congressional Budget Office. cbo.gov/sites/default/files/cbofiles/attachments/43907-BudgetOutlook.pdf. Accessed May 7, 2013.

"Nevertheless..." Roundtable discussion on "Medicare physician payments: Understanding the past so we can envision the future." finance. senate.gov/hearings/hearing/?id=ce954372-5056-a032-5269-10f65a59f5d-4May 10, 2012. Accessed October 7, 2012.

"The American Medical Association…" Letter to Sens. Max Baucus and Orrin Hatch. http://www.ama-assn.org/resources/doc/washington/sgr-transition-principles-sign-on-letter.pdf. October 15, 2012. Accessed November 12, 2012.

"In October 2013…" Medicare and the health care delivery system. MedPAC. medpac.gov/documents/Jun13_EntireReport.pdfJune 2013. Accessed October 14, 2013.

"Health-care industry groups…" America's Hospitals and Health Systems letter to Congress. *www.aha.org/advocacy-issues/letter/2012/120201-congress-halo.pdf.* February 1, 2012. Accessed February 3, 2012.

"According to the Texas Medical Association…" Medicare meltdown redux fact sheet. texmed.org/Medicare_Meltdown/. Accessed February 3, 2012.

"So far…" OIG Memorandum Report. http://oig.hhs.gov/oei/reports/oei-07-11-00340.pdf. January 26, 2012. Accessed February 2, 2012.

"In many respects…" Decker SL. In 2011 nearly one-third of physicians said they would not accept new Medicaid patients, but rising fees may help. *Health Aff.* 2012;31(8):1673-1679.

"In fact…" Gruber J, Rodriquez D. How much uncompensated care do doctors provide? NBER Working Paper 13585. http://www.nber.org/papers/w13585.pdf. November 2007. Accessed October 8, 2012.

"Under the ACA…" Foster RS. The financial outlook for Medicare, Medicaid, and total national health expenditures. Testimony before the House Committee on the Budget. budget.house.gov/uploadedfiles/fostert-estimony_2-28-22012.pdf. February 28, 2012. Accessed October 7, 2012; Shatto JD, Clemens MK. Projected Medicare expenditures under illustrative scenarios with alternative payment updates to Medicare providers. Centers for Medicare and Medicaid Services Office of the Actuary. cms.gov/Research-Statistics-Data-and-Systems/Statistics-Trends-and-Reports/ReportsTrustFunds/Downloads/2012TRAlternativeScenario.pdf. May 18, 2012. Accessed October 7, 2012; Physician practice trends survey 2012: preliminary results. Jackson Healthcare. jacksonhealthcare.com/media-room/surveys/physician-practice-trends-survey-2012.aspx. May 2012. Accessed October 7, 2012.

"Physician fees from Medicaid increased…" Zuckerman S, Williams AF, Stockley KE. Trends in Medicaid physician fees, 2003-2008. *Health Aff.*

2009;28(3):w510-W519.

CHAPTER 3

"To understand..." Auerbach DI, Kellermann AI. A decade of health care cost growth has wiped out real income gains for an average U.S. family. *Health Aff.* 2011;30(9):1630-1636.

"In less than a decade..." 2011 Milliman Medical Index: Health care costs for American families double in less than nine years. publications.milliman.com/periodicals/mmi/pdfs/milliman-medical-index-2011.pdf May 2011. Accessed May 23, 2011.

"However, more than 1..." Galbraith AA, Sinaiko AD, Soumerai SB. Some families who purchased health coverage through the Massachusetts Connector wound up with high financial burdens. *Health Aff.* 2013;32(5):974-983.

"Before the introduction of Medicare..." Baicker K, Goldman D. Patient cost-sharing and healthcare spending growth. *Journal of Economic Perspectives.* 2011;25(2):47-68; Accounting for the cost of U.S. health care: A new look at why Americans spend more. McKinsey Global Institute. mckinsey.com/mgi/publications/US_healthcare/Executive_Summary.asp. December 2008. Accessed May 24, 2011.

"Despite steeper..." National Health Expenditures 2011 Highlights. U.S. Department of Health and Human Services. cms.gov/Research-Statistics-Data-and-Systems/Statistics-Trends-and-Reports/NationalHealthExpendData/NationalHealthAccountsHistorical.html. Accessed May 29, 2013.

"A Deloitte study estimates..." The hidden costs of U.S. health care for consumers: A comprehensive analysis. Deloitte website. deloitte.com/assets/Dcom-UnitedStates/Local%20Assets/Documents/US_CHS_HiddenCostsofUSHealthCareforConsumers_032111.pdf. March 2011. Accessed May 23, 2011.

"The inability to pay medical bills..." Medical bills still top consumer woe, CR poll finds. Consumer Reports website. news.consumerreports.org/health/2011/03/medical-bill-still-top-consumer-woe-cr-poll-finds.html. March 22, 2011. Accessed May 23, 2011.

"Even more disturbing...." Kaiser Health tracking poll. kff.org/kaiser-polls/8058.cfm. March 2010. Accessed May 23, 2011.

"Nearly 6 out of 10 say..." Stremikis K, Schoen C, Fryer A. A call for change: The 2011 Commonwealth Fund survey of public views of the U.S. health system. The Commonwealth Fund. commonwealthfund.org/~/media/Files/Publications/Issue%20Brief/2011/Apr/1492_Stremikis_public_views_2011_survey_ib.pdf. April 2011. Accessed May 23, 2011.

"About 40 percent of those..." Herman PM, Rissi JJ, Walsh ME. Health insurance status, medical debt, and their impact on access to care in Arizona. *Am J Public Health*. 2011;101(8):1437-1443.

"According to an ongoing…" Cunningham PJ, Felland LE. Falling behind: Americans' access to medical care deteriorates, 2003-2007. Center for Studying Health System Change. hschange.org/CONTENT/993/. June 2008. Accessed May 23, 2011.

"Even two-thirds…" Stremikis K, op cit.

"Women experience greater…" Rustgi SD, Doty MM, Collins SR. Women at risk: Why many women are forgoing needed health care. The Commonwealth Fund. commonwealthfund.org/~/media/Files/Publications/ Issue%20Brief/2009/May/Women%20at%20Risk/PDF_1262_Rustgi_women_at_risk_issue_brief_Final.pdfMay 2009. Accessed May 23, 2011.

"*Annals of Family Medicine* researchers…" Grande D, Barg FK, Johnson S, Cannuscio CC. Life disruptions for midlife and older adults with high out-of-pocket health expenditures. *Ann Fam Med*. 2013;11:37-42.

"In a *Journal*…" Moriates C, Shah NT, Arora VM. First, do no (financial) harm. *JAMA*. 2013;310(6):577-578.

"Many studies have…" Graham JD, Potyk D, Raimi E. Hospitalists' awareness of patient charges associated with inpatient care. *J Hosp Med*. 2010;5(5):295-297.

"A survey…" Tilburt JC, Wynia MK, Sheeler RD, et al. Views of U.S. physicians about controlling health care costs. *JAMA*. 2013;310(4):380-388.

"According to the Commonwealth Fund's…" Collins SR, Robertson R, Garber T, Doty MM. Insuring the future. The Commonwealth Fund. April 2013.

"About half…" The economy and health: 10 observations. HAVAS Worldwide Health. September 2011.

"However, a majority also say…" Deloitte, op cit.

"About 1 in 10 insured Californians…" Lavarreda SA, op cit.

"The U.S. Census Bureau…" Supplemental poverty measure research. U.S. Census website. census.gov/newsroom/releases/archives/poverty/ cb11-tps44.html. Accessed April 6, 2012.

"The uninsured are especially disadvantaged …" Shortchanged by medical debt fact sheet. Families USA. amiliesusa.org/assets/pdfs/medical-debt-fact-sheet.pdf November 2009. Accessed May 23, 2011.

"Only 1 out of 8…" Chappel A. The value of health insurance: Few of the uninsured have adequate resources to pay potential hospital bills. ASPE Research Brief. May 2011.

"More than 2 out of 3…" Traub A, Ruetschlin C. The plastic safety net. demos.org/publication/plastic-safety-net. May 2012. Accessed October 10, 2012.

"The number of Americans…" Collins SR, Doty MM, Robertson R,

Garber T. Help on the horizon. The Commonwealth Fund. March 2011. Accessed October 10, 2012.

"Medical expenses contributed..." Himmelstein DJ, Thorne D, Warren E, Woolhandler S. Medical bankruptcy in the United States, 2007: Results of a national study. Himmelstein DJ, Thorne D, Warren E, Woolhandler S. Medical bankruptcy in the United States, 2007: Results of a national study 2009;122(8):741-746; Medical bills underlie 60 percent of U.S. bankruptcies: study. Reuters website. reuters.com/article/2009/06/04/us-healthcare-bankruptcy-idUSTRE5530Y020090604. June 4, 2009. Accessed May 26, 2011.

"Himmelstein also examined ..." Himmelstein DJ, Thorne D, Woolhandler S. Medical bankruptcy in Masschusetts: Has health reform made a difference? *Am J Med*. 2011;124(3):224-228.

"Besides having a better medical safety nets..." Oberlander J, White J. Public attitudes toward health care spending aren't the problem; prices are. *Health Aff*. 2009;28(5):1285-1293.

"Other researchers say..." Dranove D, Millenson ML. Medical bankruptcy: Myth versus fact. *Health Aff*. 2006;25:w74-w83.

"A study of medical financial burden..." Robertson CT, Egelhof R, Hoke M. Get sick, get out: The medical causes of home mortgage foreclosures. *Health Matrix: Journal of Law-Medicine*. 2008;18(65).

"Nearly 3 out of 4..." Retirement and health care costs weighing heavily on American's minds. Harris Interactive. harrisinteractive.com/NewsRoom/HarrisPolls/tabid/447/mid/1508/articleId/1107/ctl/ReadCustom%20Default/Default.aspx. November 5, 2012. Accessed November 15, 2012.

"A study focusing on the elderly..." Pottow JA. The rise in elder bankruptcy filings and failure of U.S. bankruptcy law. Public Law and Legal Theory Working Paper Series. University of Michigan Law School. papers.ssrn.com/sol3/papers.cfm?abstract_id=1669298 . August 2010. Accessed May 23, 2011.

"Half of Medicare..." Medicare at a glancekff.org/medicare/fact-sheet/medicare-at-a-glance-fact-sheet/. November 14, 2012. Accessed May 29, 2013.

"Medicare beneficiaries..." Medicare beneficiaries' out-of-pocket spending for health care. AARP Public Policy Institute. aarp.org/health/medicare-insurance/info-05-2012/medicare-beneficiaries-out-of-pocket-spending-for-health-care-AARP-ppi-health.html. May 2012. Accessed May 29, 2013.

"According to Fidelity Investments..." Fidelity Investments estimates couples retiring in 2010 will need $250,000 to pay medical expenses during retirement. fidelity.com/inside-fidelity/employer-services/fidelity-estimates-couple-retiring-in-2010-will-need-250000-to-cover-healthcare-costs. March 25, 2010. Accessed May 26, 2011.

"Merrill Lynch investment clients..." Merrill Lynch affluent insights survey. wealthmanagement.ml.com/wm/Pages/Affluent-Insights-Survey.aspx. February 22, 2012. Accessed April 6, 2012.

"The Center for Retirement Research..." Webb A, Zhivan N. What is the distribution of lifetime health care costs from age 65? Center for Retirement Research at Boston College website. prudential.com/media/managed/Distri_of_Lifetime_Health_Costs_from_age65.pdf March 2010. Accessed May 26, 2011.

"The price of private..." Schoen C, Lippa J, Collins S, Radley D. State trends in premiums and deductibles, 2003-2011: Eroding protection and rising costs underscore need for action. The Commonwealth Fund. December 2012.

"Large companies..." Towers Watson/NBGH employer survey on purchasing value in health care. towerswatson.com/en/Insights/IC-Types/Survey-Research-Results/2013/03/Towers-Watson-NBGH-Employer-Survey-on-Value-in-Purchasing-Health-Care. March 2013. Accessed May 29, 2013.

"One out of 3 workers..." Employer Health Benefits 2011 Annual Survey. Kaiser Family Foundation. ehbs.kff.org/. September 2011. Accessed April 6, 2012.

"A classic study..." Brook RH, Ware JE, Rogers WH, et al. *The effect of coinsurance on the health of adults: Results from the RAND Health Insurance Experiment.* Santa Monica, CA: RAND Corp. December 1984.

"A more recent study..." Chandra A; Gruber J; McKnight R. Patient cost-sharing and hospitalization offsets in the elderly. *The American Economic Review.* 2010;100(1):193-213.

"In another study..." Galbraith AA, Soumeral SB, Ross-Degnan D, Rosenthal MB, Gay C, Lieu TA. Delayed and forgone care for families with chronic conditions in high-deductible plans. J Gen Intern Medncbi.nlm.nih.gov/pubmed/22249829. January 18, 2012. Accessed April 6, 2012.

"In 2009, just 1 percent..." Cohen SB, Yu W. The concentration and persistence in the level of health expenditures over time: Estimates for the U.S. population, 2008-2009. Agency for Healthcare Research and Quality. meps.ahrq.gov/mepsweb/data_files/publications/st354/stat354.pdf. January 2012. Accessed April 6, 2012.

"Consumers do more research..." Fall 2011 Altarum Institute Center for Consumer Choice in Health Care Opinions. altarum.org/files/imce/Consumer-Choice_Fall-2011-Findings_121211.pdf. December 2011. Accessed April 6, 2012.

"A RAND Corp. study..." Haviland AM, Marquis MS, McDevitt RD, Sood N. Growth of consumer-directed health plans to one-half of all employer-sponsored insurance could save $57 billion annually. *Health Aff.* 2012;31(5):1009-1015.

"According to a National..." Large U.S. employers expect to hold health care benefit cost increases to 7 percent in 2014, National Business Group on Health Survey finds. businessgrouphealth.org/pressroom/pressRelease. cfm?ID=214. August 28, 2013. Accessed October 16, 2013.

"Companies with at least 50 percent..." Purchasing value in health care. Towers Watson website. towerswatson.com/assets/pdf/1258/WT-2010-15571.pdf. 2010. Accessed May 18, 2011.

"Nearly 25 percent..." Kullgren JT, Galbraith AA, Hinrichsen VL, et al. Health care use and decision making among lower-income families in high-deductible health plans. *Arch Intern Med.* 2010;170(21):1918-1925.

"Physician visits..." Fronstin P, Sepulveda MJ, Roebuck MC. Consumer-directed health plans reduce the long-term use of outpatient visits and prescription drugs. *Health Aff.* 2013;32(6):1126-1134.

"Access to care..." Kenney GM, ZuckermanS, Goin D, McMorrow S. Virtually every state experiencing deteriorating access to care for adults over the past decade. Urban Institute. urban.org/UploadedPDF/412560-Virtually-Every-State-Experienced-Deteriorating-Access-to-Care-for-Adults-over-th e-Past-Decade.pdf May 2012. Accessed October 11, 2012.

"For several years..." Kaiser Health Tracking Poll—May 2012. kff.org/ kaiserpolls/8315.cfmAccessed October 10, 2012.

"A 2011 recent RAND study..." Haviland AM, Sood N, McDevitt R, Marquis MS. How do consumer-directed health plans affect vulnerable populations? *Forum for Health Economics & Policy.* 2011;14(2).

"One study of health plans..." Trivedi AN, Moloo H, Mor V. Increased ambulatory care copayments and hospitalizations among the elderly. *N Engl J Med.* 2010;362(4):320-328.

"For example, high cost-sharing..." Solomon MD, Goldman DP, Joyce GF, Escarce JJ. Cost sharing and the initiation of drug therapy for the chronically ill. *Arch Intern Med.* 2009;169(8):740-748.

"For example, Pitney Bowes..." Mahoney JJ. Value-based benefit design: Using a predictive modeling approach to improve compliance. *Journal of Managed Care Pharmacy.* 2008;14(6 Suppl. B):3-8.

"A 2007 study concluded..." Goldman DP, Joyce G, Zheng. Varying pharmacy benefits with clinical status: The case of cholesterol-lowering therapy. *JAMA.* 2007;298(1):61-69.

"What is puzzling is that HDHPs..." Buntin MB, Haviland AM, McDevitt R, Sood N. Healthcare spending and preventive care in high-deductible and consumer-directed health plans. *Am J Manag Care.* 2011;17(3):222-230.

"The healthiest 50 percent..." Blumberg LJ. High-risk pools – merely a stopgap reform. *N Engl J Med.* 2011;364:e39.

"The harsh reality..." An unequal burden: The true cost of high-deductible health plans for communities of color. FamiliesUSA website. familiesusa. org/assets/pdfs/unequal-burden.pdf. September 2008. Accessed May 18,

2011.

"**A 2008 consumer survey...**" Cordina J, Singhai S. What consumers want in health care. The McKinsey Quarterly. mckinseyquarterly.com/ What_consumers_want_in_health_care_2145. June 2008. Accessed May 18, 2011.

CHAPTER 4

"**Consider:...**" Market insights: The evolution of consumer engagement in healthcare. Porter Research. 2013.

"**But only 3 percent...**" Fine LJ, Philogene GS, Gramling R, Coups EJ, Sinha S. Prevalence of multiple chronic disease risk factors. 2001 National Health Interview Survey. *Am J Prev Med.* 2004;27(2 Suppl):18-24.

"**The federal government's...**" National Center for Health Statistics Healthy People 2010 final review. Hyattsville, MD. 2012.

"**The percentage of those...**" King DE, Mainous AG, Geesy ME. Turning back the clock: Adopting a healthy lifestyle in middle age. *Am J Med.* 2007;120:598-603.

"**The National eHealth Collaborative...**" 2012 NeHC stakeholder survey results. nationalehealth.org/ckfinder/userfiles/files/2012%20NeHC%20Stakeholder%20Survey%20Results%20FINAL.pdf. 2012. Accessed October 1, 2012.

"**One study found...**" Hibbard JH, Greene J, Overton V. Patients with lower activation associated with higher costs; delivery systems should know their patients' "scores." *Health Aff.* 2013;32(2):216-222.

"**Being a compliant patient...**" Steiner JF. Rethinking adherence. *Ann Intern Med.* 2012;157:580-585.

"**In a poll...**" National Community Health Survey. atlanticlive.theatlantic.com/pr/CommunityHealth/PollResults.pdf March 2013. Accessed May 29, 2013.

"**Baby boomers are...**" King DE, Matheson E, Chirina S, Shankar A, Broman-Fulks J. The status of baby boomers' health in the United States. *JAMA Intern Med.* 2013;173(5):385-386.

"**A 2009 poll of 2,000 Americans...**" GE Better Health 2010 study fact sheet: Patient-doctor disconnect on healthy living revealed. files.healthymagination.com/wp-content/uploads/2010/02/GE-Better-Health-Study-Fact-Sheet.pdf. Accessed January 21, 2011.

"**Doctors also do not think...**" Huang J, Yu H, Marin E, Brock S, Carden D, Davis T. Physicians' weight loss counseling in two public hospital primary care clinics. *Acad Med.* 2004;79(2):156-161.

"**According to a survey...**" Foster GD, Wadden T, Makris, A et al. Primary care physicians' attitudes about obesity and its treatment. *Obes Res.*

2003;11(10):1168-1177.

"Only about one-third..." Stafford RS, Farhat JH, Misra B, Shoenfeld DA. National patterns of physician activities related to obesity management. *Arch Fam Med.* 2000;9(7):156-161.

"Barely 1 in 10 diabetics..." Eliat-Adar S, Xu J, Zephier E, O'Leary V, Howard BV, Resnick, HE. Adherence to dietary recommendations for saturated fat, fiber, and sodium is low in American Indians and other US adults with diabetes. *J Nutr.* 2008;138(9):1699-1704.

"About 18 percent of heart disease..." Soni, A. *Personal health behaviors for heart disease prevention among the US adult civilian non-institutionalized population 2004.* Rockville, MD: Agency for Healthcare Research and Quality; March 2007. MEPS statistical brief 165.

"In one study..." Calfas KJ, Long BJ, Sallis JF, Wooten WJ, Pratt M, Patrick K. A controlled trial of physician counseling to promote the adoption of physical activity. *Prev Med.* 1996;25(3):225-233.

"The American Heart Association..." Artinian NT, Fletcher GF, Mozaffarian D, et al. Interventions to promote physical activity and dietary lifestyle changes for cardiovascular risk factor reduction in adults. A scientific statement from the American Heart Association. *Circulation.* 2010;122:406-441.

"There is a misguided belief..." Puhl RM, Brownell KD. Confronting and coping with weight stigma: An investigation of overweight and obese adults. *Obesity.* 2006;(14)10:1802-1815.

"Examples of weight bias do not get..." Pomeranz JL. A historical analysis of public health, the law, and stigmatized social groups: The need for both obesity and weight bias legislation. *Obesity.* 2008;16:S93-S102.

"Studies consistently show..." Saban JA, Marini M, Nosek BA. Implicit and explicit anti-fat bias among a large same of medical doctors by BMI, race/ethnicity and gender. *PLOS One.* November 2012;(7)11:e48448.

"There even is..." Miller DP, Spangler JG, Vitolins MZ, et al. Are medical students aware of their anti-obesity bias? *Acad Med.* 2013;88(7):978-82.

"In a study..." Gudzune KA, Beach MC, Roter DL, Cooper LA. Physicians build less rapport with obese patients. *Obesity.* 2013. DOI: 10.1002/oby.20384. Accessed June 3, 2013.

"Overweight or obese..." Gudzune KA, Bleich SN, Richards TM. Doctor shopping by overweight and obese patients is association with increased healthcare utilization. *Obesity.* onlinelibrary.wiley.com/doi/10.1002/oby.20189/abstract May 13, 2013. Accessed June 7, 2013.

"Healthier physicians apparently..." Frank E, Dresner Y, Shani M, Vinker S. The association between physicians' and patients' preventive health practices. *CMAJ.* 2013;185(8):649-653.

"Researchers reviewed..." Garcia I, Lobelo F. Healthcare providers as role models for physical activity. 2013 American Heart Association Epidemiology and Prevention/Nutrition, Physical Activity and Metabolism conference, New Orleans, LA; abstract P420.

"U.S. physicians...." Bass K., McGeeney K. U.S. physicians set good health example. Gallup. October 3, 2013.

"Physicians can lose..." Puhl RM, Gold JA, Luedicke J, Depierre JA. The effect of physicians' body weight on patient attitudes: implications for physician selection, trust and adherence to medical advice. *Int J Obes*. ncbi.nlm.nih.gov/pubmed/23507996. March 19, 2013. Accessed May 29, 2013; Yancey AK, Sallis RF, Bastani. Changing physical activity participation for the medical profession. *JAMA*. 2013;309(2):141-142.

"Only half of those..." Naderi SH, Bestwick JP, Wald DS. Adherence to drugs that prevent cardiovascular disease: Meta-analysis on 376,162 patients. *Am J Med*. 201;125(9):882-7

"An extreme example is..." Smokers refused operations. TVNZ. tvnz.co.nz/content/28552/425826.html. February 8, 2001. Accessed February 8, 2010.

"At least 40 percent of smokers..." Ulene V. Why are unhealthy people so reluctant to change their lifestyles? *The Los Angeles Times*. May 23, 2011.

"One out of 5..." Weaver KE, Rowland JH, Augustson E, Atienza AA. Smoking concordance in lung and colorectal cancer patient-caregiving dyads and quality of life. *Cancer Epidemiol Biomarkers Prevent*. 2011;20:239-248.

"Consultant Leonard Kish..." Kish L. The blockbuster drug of the century: An engaged patient. hl7standards.com/blog/2012/08/28/drug-of-the-century/. August 28, 2012. Accessed October 14, 2013.

"How many do this?...." Snapshot of people's engagement in their health care. Center for Advancing Health. cfah.org/activities/snapshot.cfm. May 20, 2010. Accessed May 2, 2011.

"Engaged patients are not..." Hibbard JH, Stockard J, Mahoney ER, Tusler, M. Development of the Patient Activation Measure (PAM): Conceptualizing and measuring activation in patients and consumers. *Health Serv Res*. 2004;39(4 Pt 1):1005-1026.

"Consider that physicians spend..." Choice in medical care: When should the consumer decide? Academy Health website. academyhealth.org/files/issues/ConsumerDecide.pdf. October 2007. Accessed May 4, 2011.

"They forget 40 to 80 percent..." Kessels, RP. Patients' memory for medical information. *J R Soc Med*. 2003;96(5):219-222.

"Six out of 10..." Jammed access: Widening the front door to healthcare. PricewaterhouseCoopers website. pwc.com/us/en/healthcare/publications/jammed-access-widening-the-front-door-to-healthcare.jhtml. July 2009. Accessed May 2, 2011.

"Researcher Judith Hibbard..." Hibbard J. Engaging consumers to improve health and reduce costs. Presentation, Alliance for Health Reform. March 5, 2010.

"Hibbard found that..." Greene J, Hibbard JH, Sacks R, Overton V. When seeing the same physician, highly activated patients have better care experiences than less activated patients. *Health Aff.* 2013;32(7):1295-1305.

"The typical health consumer..." Center for Advancing Health, op. cit.

"The American Medical Association ..." Kon, AA. The shared decision-making continuum. *JAMA.* 2010;304(8):903-904.

"Patients make a large numbeR..." Wennberg D, Barbeau B, Gerry E. Power to the Patient: The importance of shared decision-making. Health Dialog website. resources.healthdialog.com/Power-to-the-Patient-Research. html. June 2009. Accessed May 2, 2011.

"One study found a 20 to 30 percent reduction..." O'Connor A, Stacey D, Entwistle V, et al. Decision aids for people facing health treatment or screening decisions. *Cochrane Database Syst Rev.* 2003. (2):CD001431.

"There are other benefits..." Crawford M, Rutter D, Manley C, et al. Systematic review of involving patients in the planning and development of health care. *BMJ.* 2002;325:1263-1266.

"A study of nine common medical decisions..." Zikmund-Fisher, Couper MP, Singer E, et al. The DECISIONS Study: A nationwide survey of United States adults regarding 9 common medical decisions. *Med Decis Making.* 2010:30(5 suppl.): 20S-34S.

"The American Heart Association..." Allen LA, Stevenson LW, Grady KI. Decision making in advanced heart failure: A scientific statement from the American Heart Association. circ.ahajournals.org/content/125/15/1928 March 5, 2012. Accessed October 1, 2012.

"One clear barrier..." Adams JR, Legare F, Frosch DL. Communicating with physicians about medical decisions: A reluctance to disagree. *Arch Intern Med.* 2012;172(15):1184-1186.

"In a *Health Affairs* study..." Frosch DL, May SG, Rendel KAS, Tietbohl C, Elwyn G. Authoritarian physicians and patients' fear of being labeled 'difficult' among key obstacles to shared decision making. *Health Aff.* 2012;31(5):1030-1038.

"Physician-patient discussions..." Braddock CH, Edwards KA, Hasenberg NM, Laidley TL, Levinson W. Informed decision making in outpatient practice. *JAMA.* 1999;282(24):2313-2320.

"Nearly all patients..." Sarasohn-Kahn J. Consumerism growing in health care, says Altarum. healthpopuli.com/2012/09/14/consumerism-growing-in-health-care-says-altarum/September 14, 2012. Accessed October 1, 2012.

"Dr. Google..." Fox S, Duggan M. Health online 2013. Pew Research

Center. pewinternet.org/Reports/2013/Health-online.aspx. January 15, 2013. Accessed April 17, 2013.

"A separate survey…" Survey: Consumers show high degree of trust in online health information, report success in self-diagnosis. Wolters Kluwer Health. wolterskluwerhealth.com/News/Pages/Survey-Consumers-Show-High-Degree-of-Trust-in-Online-Health-Information,-Report-Success-in-Self-Diagnosis--.aspx May 16, 2012. Accessed April 17, 2013.

"One out of 2 patients…" Health reform – prospering in a post-reform world. PricewaterhouseCoopers website. pwc.com/us/en/health-industries/publications/prospering-in-a-post-reform-world.jhtml. May, 2010. Accessed May 2, 2011; The customization of diagnosis, care and cure. pwc.com/us/en/healthcast/index.jhtml?wt.ac=healthindustries_healthcast. May 2010. Accessed May 11, 2011

"In fact, seeking health information…" Fox, S. 80% of Internet users look for health information online. Pew Research Center website. http://www.pewinternet.org/Reports/2011/HealthTopics.aspx. February 1, 2011. Accessed May 2, 2011.

"Avid users…" "Cyberchondriacs" on the rise? Harris Interactive website. harrisinteractive.com/NewsRoom/HarrisPolls/tabid/447/mid/1508/articleId/448/ctl/ReadCustom%20Default/Default.aspx. August 4, 2010. Accessed May 2, 2011.

"The most frequent reasons…" McDaid D, Park A. Online health: Untangling the Web. Bupa website. bupa.com/jahia/webdav/site/bupacom/shared/Documents/PDFs/media-centre/Health%20Pulse%20-%20HW/Online%20Health%20-%20Untangling%20the%20Web.pdf. January 4, 2011. Accessed May 2, 2011.

"More than half who sought…" Tu HT, Cohen GR. Striking jump in consumers seeking health care information. Center for Studying Health System Changehschange.org/CONTENT/1006/. August 2008. Accessed May 2, 2011.

"Researchers reviewed 343 website pages…" Bernstam EV, Walji MF, Sagaram S, et al. Commonly cited website quality criteria are not effective at identifying inaccurate online information about breast cancer. *Cancer.* 2008;112(6):1206-1213.

"A 2009 poll found…" Kaiser Health tracking poll: 2009. kff.org/kaiser-polls/upload/7944.pdf. Accessed May 11, 2011.

"Dr. Michael Fisch…" Parker-Pope T. You're sick. Now what? Knowledge is power. *The New York Times,* September 30, 2008.

"Most U.S. adults still trust…" Fox, S. Mobile Health 2010. PewResearchCenter website. pewinternet.org/Reports/2010/Mobile-Health-2010.aspx. October 19, 2010. Accessed May 2, 2011.

"About 70 percent of patients…" Hu X, Bell RA, Kravitz R, Orrange S.

The prepared patient: Information seeking of online support group members before their medical appointment. *Journal of Health Communication.* 2012;17(8):960-978.

"However, a 2012 Wolters Kluwer..." Survey: Consumers show high degree of trust in online health information, report success in self-diagnosis. Wolters Kluwer. wolterskluwerhealth.com/News/Pages/Survey-Consumers-Show-High-Degree-of-Trust-in-Online-Health- Information,-Report-Success-in-Self-Diagnosis--.aspx. May 16, 2012. Survey: Physicians see improvements in efficiency, quality of care, yet significant barriers remain. wolterskluwerhealth.com/News/Pages/Survey-Physicians-See-Improvements-in-Efficiency,-Quality-of-Care,-Yet-Significant-Barriers-Remain.aspx. November 1, 2011. Accessed October 1, 2012.

"Physicians are required..." Delbanco T, Walker J, Bell SK, et al. Inviting patients to read their doctors' notes: A quasi-experimental study and a look ahead. Ann Intern Med. 2012;157:461-470.

"Physicians are shying away..." Patient survey: Docs silent on health

CHAPTER 5

"In 2001..." The ballot or the wallet. Policy prescription blog. policyprescriptions.org/the-ballot-or-the-wallet/. August 27, 2012. Accessed November 1, 2012; Grande D, Asch DA, Armstrong K. Do doctors vote? *J Gen Intern Med.* 2007;22:565-569.

"In Deloitte's ..." 2013 Deloitte survey of U.S. physicians. deloitte.com/view/en_US/us/Insights/centers/center-for-health-solutions/a5ee019120e6d-310VgnVCM1000003256f70aRCRD.htm?id=us_furl_2013physciansurvey_031813. Accessed April 30, 2013.

"However, two-thirds of physicians ..." Survey findings: Physician attitudes on the Affordable Care Act. Jackson Healthcare. jacksonhealthcare.com/media-room/surveys/physician-attitudes-on-the-affordable-care-act-2012.aspx. Accessed November 1, 2012.

"Younger and prospective ..." Sommers BD, Bindman AB. New physicians, the Affordable Care Act, and the changing practice of medicine. *JAMA.* 2012;307(16):1697-1698.

"Yet a Physicians Foundation ..." 2012 Great American physician survey data. physicianspractice.com/great-american-physician-survey/2012-great-american-physician-survey-data. September 4, 2012. Accessed November 1, 2012.

"To understand ..." Kaiser Health Tracking Poll: April 2013. kff.org/health-reform/poll-finding/kaiser-health-tracking-poll-april-2013/. April 30, 2013. Accessed June 4, 2013.

"Most Americans ..." InsuranceQuotes.com survey: Many Americans fail to grasp health care form. insurancequotes.com/health-care-reform-law/#.

UYAJQMoWSXI. Accessed April 30, 2013.

"Physicians are shying away ..." Patient survey: Docs silent on health reform. HealthPocket. July 2, 2013. prnewswire.com/news-releases/patient-survey-docs-silent-on-health-reform-213974141.html. Accessed October 9, 2013; Kaiser Health tracking poll: August 2013. kff.org/health-reform/poll-finding/kaiser-health-tracking-poll-august-2013/. Accessed October 9, 2013.

"More than half ..." Physicians in the dark about how health insurance exchanges work. LocumTenens.com. locumtenens.com/press-releases/2013-archive/physicians-in-the-dark-about-how-health-insurance-exchanges-will-work.aspx. Accessed October 9, 2013.

"According to a Medical..." Pittman D. Docs skeptical of ACA exchanges survey shows. *MedPage Today.* October 7, 2013.

"This process unduly..." Letter to Marilyn Tavenner. op.bna.com/hl.nsf/id/stee-9amre3/$File/MHA-MSMA%20Joint%20ltr%20copy%20%283%29.pdf. August 12, 2013. Accessed November 26, 2013.

"Urban Institute researchers..." Zukerman S, Berenson R. How will physicians be affected by health care reform? Urban Institute. July 2010.

"Ezekiel Emanuel..." Pittman D. Docs told they must drive health system change. Medpage Today. April 11, 2013.

"Two University of Pennsylvania..." Asch DA, Volpp KG. What is the business of health care? *Harvard Business Review.* blogs.hbr.org/cs/2012/09/what_is_the_business_of_health.htmlSeptember 13, 2012 Accessed October 9, 2012.

"Richard Foster..." Foster RS. The financial outlook for Medicare, Medicaid, and total national health expenditures. Testimony before the House Committee on the Budget. February 28, 2012.

"Medical practices..." MGMA-ACPME. 2012 payer study results. mgma.com/WorkArea/DownloadAsset.aspx?id=1372690 Accessed December 10, 2012.

"The National Commission..." The National Commission on Physician Payment Reform. physicianpaymentcommission.org/report/; physicianpaymentcommission.org/press/March 4, 2013. Accessed April 28, 2013.

"About 1 out of 3..." Bundled Care. Booz & Co. booz.com/media/file/BoozCo_Bundled-Care-Employers-Payors.pdf. Accessed November 21, 2013.

"Physicians stand..." Duszak R, Burleson J, Seidenwurm, Silva E. Medicare's physician quality reporting system: Early national radiologist experience and near-future performance projections. *Journal of the American College of Radiology.* 2013;10(2):114-121.

"Another threat is..." hlc.org/blog/wp-content/uploads/2013/04/IPAB-Group-Letter-April-25-20131.pdf; hlc.org/2013/04/over-500-organizations-representing-patients-healthcare-providers-employers-urge-congress-to-eliminate-ipab/#more-10131.

"Regardless of all..." catalyzepaymentreform.org/images/documents/release.pdf. March 26, 2013. Accessed April 29, 2013; Farewell to fee-for-service? UnitedHealth Center for Health Reform & Modernization. December 2010.

"The risk..." Ter Matt, S. Medical directors' duties linked to quality metrics. *American Medical News.* May 7, 2013. Accessed June 4, 2013.

"A UnitedHealth Group..." Kulkarni SS. Report: Payment reform leaves docs uneasy. Kaiser Health News. December 10, 2012.

"However, 9 out of 10..." Deloitte 2013 survey of U.S. physicians. deloitte.com/assets/Dcom-UnitedStates/Local%20Assets/Documents/us_chs_2013SurveyofUSPhysicians_031813.pdf. Accessed June 7, 2013.

"According to an MGMA survey..." Medical practice executives cite financial management issues as most challenging. MGMA. June 25, 2013. mgma.com/press/default.aspx?id=1374836. Accessed October 8, 2013

"A Robert Wood Johnson Foundation essay..." Painter MW. Improving incentives. Robert Wood Johnson Foundation. August 7, 2013.

"A *Cochrane Collaboration* review..." Scott A, Sivey P, Ouakrim DA, et al. The effect of financial incentives on the quality of health care provided by primary care physicians. *The Cochrane Collaboration.* September 7, 2011. onlinelibrary.wiley.com/doi/10.1002/14651858.CD008451.pub2/abstract;jsessionid=1D64A0B4D818A6CC464BDC968280478D.d01t04. Accessed October 9, 2013.

"Remarkably, about 1 out of 4..." 2013 Physician Sentiment Index. athenahealth. athenahealth.com/physician-sentiment-index/_doc/2013_Physician_Sentiment_Index.pdf. Accessed October 8, 2013.

"Health-care executives..." Getting from volume to value in health care. Forbes Insights. images.forbes.com/forbesinsights/StudyPDFs/AllscriptsVolumetoValue.pdf. May 14, 2012. Accessed June 4, 2013.

"ACOs spread swiftly..." Accountable care organizations now serve 14 percent of Americans. reuters.com/article/2013/02/19/ny-oliver-wyman-idUS-nBwb7Y0jya+110+BSW20130219 February 19, 2013. Accessed April 30, 2013.

"David Mulestein..." Muhlestein D. Why has ACO growth slowed? *Health Affairs* blog. healthaffairs.org/blog/2013/10/31/why-has-aco-growth-slowed/. October 31, 2013.

"Nonetheless, ACOs are expected..." Health plan readiness to operationalize new payment models. Availity. availity.com/news-resources/case-studies/. Accessed June 4, 2013.

"ACOs now treat..." Gandhi N, Weil R. The ACO surprise. Oliver Wyman. oliverwyman.com/the-aco-surprise.htm#.UMTr84awW_k November 2012. Accessed December 10, 2012.

"More than half..." Lowes R. SGR jitters deter physicians from new Medicare pay models. *Medscape.* October 23, 2012.

"Nearly 2 out of 3..." Spoerl B. 63% of physicians say ACOs will have negative impact on care. beckershospitalreview.com/hospital-physician-relationships/63-of-physicians-say-acos-will-have-negative-impact-on-care.html June 14, 2012. Accessed November 1, 2012.

"The number ..." Physician compensation report 2013. *Medscape.* medscape.com/features/slideshow/compensation/2013/public. Accessed April 30, 2013.

"About 4 out of 10..." Accountable to whom? LocumTenens.com. locumtenens.com/media/81064/accountable_care-final.pdf. Accessed April 30, 2013.

"Paul Ginsburg..." Pittman D. Doc-led ACOs better model for saving $$$. *Medpage Today.* May 15, 2013.

"Of those choosing..." Muhlestein D, Croshaw A, Merrill T, Pena C. Growth and dispersion of accountable care organizations: June 2012 update. Leavitt Partners. leavittpartners.com/wp-content/uploads/2012/06/Growth-and-Dispersion-of-ACOs-June-2012-Update.pdfAccessed November 1, 2012.

"Regardless of whether..." Huang G. 5 ways ACOs will impact your practice even if you don't participate. pbn.decisionhealth.com/Articles/Detail.aspx?id=512365 . May 7, 2012. Accessed November 1, 2012.

"Despite the proliferation..." Noble DJ, Casalino LP. Can accountable care organizations improve population health? *JAMA.* 2013;309(11):1119-1120.

"ACOs that improved..." Eddy DM, Shah R. A simulation shows limited savings from meeting quality targets under the Medicare Shared Savings Program. *Health Aff.* October 11, 2012. Accessed November 1, 2012; Audet A, Kenward K, Patel S, Joshi, M. Hospitals on the path to accountable care: Highlights from a 2011 National Survey of Hospital Readiness to Participate in an Accountable Care Organization. The Commonwealth Fund. commonwealthfund.org/Publications/Issue-Briefs/2012/Aug/Hospitals-on-the-Path-to-Accountable-Care.aspxAugust 2012. Accessed November 6, 2012.

"Researchers Lawton Burns..." Burns LR, Pauly MV. Accountable care organizations may have difficulty avoiding the failures of integrated delivery networks of the 1990s. *Health Aff.* 2012;31(11):2412-2416.

"Compared with ACOs..." Nielsen M, Langer B, Zema C, Hacker T, Grundy P. Benefits of implementing the primary care patient-centered medical home: A review of cost & quality results, 2012. Patient-Centered Primary

Care Collaborative. pcpcc.net/guide/benefits-implementing-pcmh. Accessed November 1, 2012.

"A WellPoint pilot..." Raskas RS, Latts LM, Hummel JR, Wenners D, Levine H, Nussbaum SR. Early results show Wellpoint's patient-centered medical home pilots have met some goals for costs, utilization, and quality. *Health Aff.* 2012;31(9):2002-2009.

"PCMHs are given..." Fifield J, Forrest DD, Martin-Pelle M, et al. A randomized, controlled trial of implementing the patient-centered medical home model in solo and small practices. *J Gen Intern Med.* ncbi.nlm.nih.gov/pubmed/22956444. September 7, 2012. Accessed November 6, 2012.

"CareFirst BlueCross..." Sun LH. CareFirst says experimental program improves primary care, reduces costs. *The Washington Post.* June 7, 2012.

"Studies have questioned..." Jackson GL, Powers BJ, Chatterjee R, et al. The patient-centered medical home: A systematic review. *Ann Intern Med.* 2013;158(3):169-178; Peikes D, Zutshi A, Genevro JL, et al. Early evaluations of the medical home: Building on a promising start. Am J Manag Care. 2012;18(2):105-116.

" A survey of more than 1,300..." Martsolf GR, Alexander JA, Shi Y, et al. The patient-centered medical home and patient experience. *Health Serv Res.* ncbi.nlm.nih.gov/pubmed/22670806June 7, 2012. Accessed November 6, 2012; O'Reilly KB. Shift to medical home may not increase patient satisfaction. American Medical News. July 2, 2012.

"From a physician's perspective..." Nocon RS, Sharma R, Birnberg JM, et al. Association between patient-centered medical home rating and operating cost at federally funded health centers. *JAMA.* 2012;308(1):60-66; Reid RJ, Larson EB. Financial implications of the patient-centered medical home. JAMA. 2012;308(1):83-84.

"A federally funded ..." Jackson GL, Powers BJ, Chatterjee R, et al. The patient-centered medical home: A systematic review. *Ann Intern Med.* annals.org/article.aspx?articleid=1402441November 27, 2012. Accessed December 10, 2012.

"The Patient Centered..." PCPCC leadership responds to latest medical home "systematic review." pcpcc.org/sites/default/files/media/Press%20Release%20-%20PCPCC%20Statement%20on%20Systematic%20Review%20-%2012-3-12.pdf. Accessed December 10, 2012.

"The federal government..." Doctors and hospitals' use of health IT more than doubles in 2012. U.S. Department of Health and Human Services. hhs.gov/news/press/2013pres/05/20130522a.htmlMay 22, 2013. Accessed May 30, 2013.

"Despite the fact..." DesRoches CM, Audet A, Painter M, Donelan. Meaningful use criteria and managing patient populations. Ann Intern Med. 2013;158(11):791-799; Koppel R. Demanding utility from health information technology. *Ann Intern Med.* 2013;158(11):845-846.

"Nearly 1 out of 3..." Electronic health record sellers face make-or-break year of client ultimatums and revolts, reveals 2013 Black Book survey. February 18, 2013. Accessed May 30, 2013.

"The average physician..." Doctors who adopt electronic health records may lose money. University of Michigan News Service. ns.umich.edu/new/multimedia/videos/21256-doctors-who-adopt-electronic-health-records-may-lose-money March 4, 2013. Accessed May 30, 2013.

"A county hospital ..." Lowes R. Residents skip lectures to catch up on EHR charting. *Medscape.* October 14, 2013.

CHAPTER 6

"In 1994..." Testimony of Dr. Louis McIntyre, Small Business Committee, U.S. House of Representatives. smallbusiness.house.gov/uploaded-files/7-19_mcintyre_testimony.pdf July 19, 2012. Accessed November 28, 2013.

"According to a poll by Sermo..." Ledue C. Survey: Over 26 percent of solo docs may close their practices. *Healthcare Finance News.* February 18, 2010.

"According to QuantiaMD..." Struggling primary care physicians could undermine Affordable Care Act. Quantia MD. quantiamd.com/home/pr_struggling_primary_careJuly 31, 2012. Accessed October 9, 2012.

"One out of 3 physicians..." Physician practice trends survey 2012: Preliminary results. Jackson Healthcare. jacksonhealthcare.com/media-room/surveys/physician-practice-trends-survey-2012.aspx. Accessed October 8, 2012.

"More than 75 percent..." 2012 review of physician recruiting incentives. Merritt Hawkins. merritthawkins.com/uploadedFiles/MerrittHawkins/Pdf/mha-2012survpreview.pdf. Accessed October 9, 2012.

"The share of physicians..." Clinical transformation: Dramatic changes as physician employment grows. Accenture. accenture.com/SiteCollection-Documents/PDF/Accenture_Clinical_Transformation.pdf. 2011. Accessed October 9, 2012.

"An outlier survey..." Kane CK, Emmons DW. New data on physician practice arrangements: Private practice remains strong despite shifts toward hospital employment. American Hospital Association. 2013. ama-assn.org/resources/doc/health-policy/prp-physician-practice-arrangements.pdf. Accessed October 14, 2013.

"Granted, more than 80 percent..." A roadmap for physicians to health care reform. Physicians Foundation. physiciansfoundation.org/uploaded-Files/Roadmap%20for%20Physicians%20Final%20%282%29.pdf. May 2011. Accessed April 13, 2012.

"Only 1 out of 4 physicians..." Health reform and the decline of physician private practice. The Physicians Foundation. physiciansfoundation.org/uploadedFiles/Survey%20Key%20Findings%20Nov%202010.pdf. November 2010. Accessed April 13, 2012.

"One of the demographic..." 2011 state physician workforce data book. Association of American Medical Colleges Center for Workforce Studies. aamc.org/download/263512/data/statedata2011.pdf. November 2011. Accessed March 21, 2012.

"However, more than half..." Jackson & Coker retirement study. jacksoncoker.com/documents/jcretirement_survey.pdf. August 2, 2011. Accessed April 13, 2012.

"The percentage of physicians..." Clinical transformation: Dramatic changes as physician employment grows. Accenture. accenture.com. March 28, 2011. Accessed April 16, 2012; Clinical transformation: New business models for a new era in healthcare. Accenture. accenture.com/SiteCollectionDocuments/PDF/Accenture-Clinical-Transformation-New-Business-Models-for-a-New-Era-in-Healthcare.pdf#zoom=50. October 30, 2012. Accessed December 10, 2012.

"In a 2011 survey..." Betbeze P. Physician alignment: The collaborative care disconnect. HealthLeaders Media. healthleadersmedia.com/intelligence/091/industry-insight-report.html. September 2011. Accessed April 13, 2012.

"Moreover, third-year medical residents..." 2011 Survey of Final-Year Medical Residents. Merritt Hawkins & Associates. October 5, 2011.

"According to the Medical Group Management Association..." Caffarini K. 5 simple ways to cut medical practice costs. *American Medical News*. January 9, 2012.

"An MGMA survey showed..." Cost survey for multispecialty practices: 2011 report based on 2010 data. Medical Group Management Association. mgma.com/store/Surveys-and-Benchmarking/Cost-Survey-for-Multispecialty-Practices-2011-Report-Based-on-2010-Data-Print-Edition/. 2011. Accessed April 16, 2012.

"There were more..." Health care M&A spending falls nearly 40% in 2012, lowest year on record since 2003, according to Irving Levin Associates, Inc. businesswire.com/news/home/20130121005788/en/Health-Care-MA-Spending-Falls-40-2012 January 21, 2013. Accessed November 4, 2013.

"According to a survey..." Hospitals to increase physician practice acquisitions this year. Jackson Healthcare. jacksonhealthcare.com/media-room/news/hospital-physician-practice-acquisitions-2012-2013.aspx. Accessed April 15, 2013.

"Even though Moody's..." Ter Matt, S. Moody's: Doctor integration vital to stronger hospital finances. *American Medical News*. February 11, 2013.

"More than half…" Trend watch: Physician practice acquisitions 2012-2013. Jackson Healthcare. jacksonhealthcare.com/media-room/surveys/trend-watch-physician-practice-acquisitions-2012-2013.aspx Accessed June 4, 2013.

"Physicians believe hospital employment…" PwC. From courtship to marriage, Part II. pwc.com/us/en/health-industries/publications/from-court-ship-to-marriage-series.jhtml. April 2011.

"Acquiring and integrating…" ACPE poll finds physician integration may increase costs. American College of Physician Executivesprnewswire.com/news-releases/acpe-poll-finds-physician-integration-may-increase-costs-214586931.html July 8, 2013. Accessed October 14, 2013.

"A Healthcare Financial…" HFMA's executive survey on hospital-physician affiliation. hfma.org/hospital-physicianaffiliation/. June 14, 2013. Accessed October 14, 2013.

"Hospitals also are…" Decade in review: Hospital M&A deal volume increases. Irving Levin Associates. levinassociates.com/pr2012/pr1202hospital. February 28, 2012. Accessed October 9, 2012. Brown TC, Werling KA, Walker BC, Burgdorfer RJ, Shields JJ. Current trends in hospital mergers and acquisitions. Healthc Financ Manage. 2012;66(3):114-118.

"According to Harvard economist…" Cutler DM, Morton FS. Hospitals, market share and consolidation. *JAMA*. 2013;310(18):1964-1970.

"HFMA identified…" Wilson B. Four principles to guide successful physician integration. Grant Thornton. grantthornton.com/portal/site/gtcom/menuitem.8f5399f6096d695263012d28633841ca/?vgnextoid=63dbab-6951316310VgnVCM1000003a8314acRCRD. Spring 2012. Accessed October 9, 2012.

"Cleveland Clinic President…" Betbeze P. Consolidation comes with benefits (and costs). *HealthLeaders Media*. October 14, 2013.

"A Robert Wood Johnson…" Gaynor M, Town R. The impact of hospital consolidation—update. Robert Wood Johnson Foundation. rwjf.org/content/rwjf/en/research-publications/find-rwjf-research/2012/06/the-impact-of-hospital-consolidation.html. June 2012. Accessed October 9, 2012.

"Karen Ignagni…" Creswell J, Abelson R. New laws and rising costs create a surge of supersizing hospitals. *The New York Times*. August 12, 2013.

"The resulting cost increases…" Ohlhaussen, M. Hospital consolidation: "The good, the bad and the ugly." Federal Trade Commission. ftc.gov/speeches/ohlhausen/130313hospitalconsolidationspeech.pdfMarch 13, 2013. Accessed November 4, 2013.

"By 2006…" Gaynor M. Testimony before the Committee on Ways and Means Health Subcommittee, U.S. House of Representatives. September 9,

2011.

"Consulting firm..." Succeeding in hospital and health systems M&A. Booz & Co. booz.com/media/uploads/BoozCo_Succeeding-in-Hospital-and-Health-Systems-MA.pdf. Accessed December 20, 2013

"Health reform..." The Massachusetts experience: Reform shifts the healthcare landscape. PwC. pwc.com/us/massachusettshealthreform. Accessed October 14, 2013.

"After initially knocking..." Elliott VS. Employing more physicians stabilizes hospital finances. *American Medical News.* September 12, 2012.

"A Wall Street Journal report..." Mathews AW. Same doctor visit, double the cost. *The Wall Street Journal.* August 26, 2012.

"For Merritt Hawkins..." 2012 Review of physician recruiting incentives. merritthawkins.com/uploadedFiles/MerrittHawkins/pdf/mha2012survpreview.pdf. Accessed April 13, 2013.

"One reason..." A survey of America's physicians: Practice patterns and perspectives. physiciansfoundation.org/uploads/default/Physicians_Foundation_2012_Biennial_Survey.pdf. 2012. Accessed April 13, 2013.

"Hospitals are recruiting..." Elliott VS. Many hospitals recruiting doctors continually. *American Medical News.* September 10, 2012.

"The percentage of cardiologists..." New American College of Cardiology practice census shows continued trend towards hospital integration. cardiosource.org/News-Media/Media-Center/News-Releases/2012/09/Leg-Conf.aspx. Accessed December 10, 2012.

"Physicians who become..." Ericksson physician search 2012 annual survey.ericksson.net/surveys/ErickssonSurvey.pdf. Accessed November 15, 2012; Struggling primary care physicians could undermine Affordable Care Act. quantiamd.com/home/pr_struggling_primary_care. July 31, 2012. Accessed November 16, 2012.

"More than half..." Ter Matt S. Physicians get many job overtures and should brace for more. *American Medical News.* July 8, 2013.

"The AMA House..." AMA principles for physician employment. ama-assn.org/resources/doc/hod/ama-principles-for-physician-employment.pdf. Accessed November 15, 2012.

"Hospitals and health systems..." Rodak S. 11 hospital, health system executive compensation trends. *Becker's Hospital Review.* May 8, 2012.

"The use of employment contracts ..." haygroup.com/us/press/details.aspx?id=35150. Nov. 27, 2012. Accessed April 10, 2013.

"Physician turnover..." Physician turnover hits new high as housing and stock markets recover. prnewswire.com/news-releases-test/physician-turnover-hits-new-high-as-housing-and-stock-markets-recover-198826841.html. March 18, 2013. Accessed April 15, 2013.

"According to Dr. Roger…" Kocher R, Sahni BS. Hospitals' race to employ physicians – the logic behind a losing proposition. *N Engl J Med.* 2011;364:1790-1793.

"As American Enterprise…" Gottlieb S. The doctor won't see you now. *The Wall Street Journal.* March 14, 2013.

"One health insurer…" How competitive are state insurance markets?" Kaiser Family Foundation. Focus on health reform. No. 8242. October 2011.

"A similar 2012 analysis…" New AMA study finds anticompetitive market conditions are common across managed care plans." American Medical Association. ama-assn.org/ama/pub/news/news/2012-11-28-study-finds-anticompetitive-market-conditions-common.page November 28, 2012. Accessed November 5, 2013.

CHAPTER 7

"The National Health Care Workforce…" Cheney K. The invisible health-care panel. *Politico.* January 30, 2013.

"The Congressional Budget Office…" Hanchate AD, Lasser KE, Kapoor A, Rosen J, McCormick D, D'Amore MM, et al. Massachusetts reform and disparities in inpatient care utilization. Med Care. 2012;50(7):569–77; Decker SL, Kostova D, Kenne GM, Long SK. Health status, risk factors, and medical conditions among persons enrolled in Medicaid vs. uninsured low-income adults potentially eligible for Medicaid under the Affordable Care Act. *JAMA.* 2013;309(24):2579-2586.

"Policy researchers…" Hofer AN, Abraham JM, Moscovice I. Expansion of coverage under the Patient Protection and Affordable Care Act and primary care utilization. Milbank Q. 2011;89(1):69–89; Petterson SM, Liaw WR, Phillips RL, Rabin DL, Meyers DS, Bazemore AW. Projecting U.S. primary care physician workforce needs: 2010–2025. *Ann Fam Med.* 2012;10(6):503–9.

"Their average work week…" Staiger DO, Auerbach DI, Buerhaus PI. Trends in the work hours of physicians in the United States. *JAMA.* 2010;303(8):747-753.

"Only 1 out of 4 say…" Health reform and the decline of physician private practice. The Physicians Foundation website. physiciansfoundation.org/uploadedFiles/Health%20Reform%20and%20the%20Decline%20of%20Physician%20Private%20Practice.pdf. October 2010. Accessed May 11, 2011

"The recession prompted…" Commins J. Healthcare workers delaying retirement. *Health Leaders Media.* healthleadersmedia.com/page-1/TEC-266573/Healthcare-Workers-Delaying-Retirement. May 25, 2011. Accessed July 28, 2011.

"Most experts point to…" Peterson SM, Liaw WR, Phillips RL, Rabin

DL, Meyers DS, Bazemore AW. Projecting U.S. primary care physician workforce needs: 2010-2025. *Ann Fam Med*. 2012;10(6):503-509.

"The number of those..." Dall TM, Gallo PD, Chakrabarti R, et al. An aging population and growing disease burden will require a large and specialized health care workforce by 2025. *Health Aff*. 2013;32(11):2013-2020.

"Even safety-net physicians..." Newly insured may have trouble finding primary care physicians. massgeneral.org/about/pressrelease.aspx?id=1525. November 26, 2012. Accessed December 5, 2012.

"About half..." Guila R. Massachusetts Medical Society releases 2012 patient access to care study. massmed.org/AM/Template.cfm?Section=News_and_Publications2&TEMPLATE=/CM/ContentDisplay.cfm&CONTENTID=74723. August 8, 2012. Accessed October 1, 2012.

"More than 1..." Medscape 2012 survey results. medscape.com/features/slideshow/public/ethics2012#10. Accessed May 29, 2013.

"According to a *JAMA*..." Michtalik HJ, Yeh H, Pronovost PJ, Brotman DJ. Impact of attending physician workload on patient care: A survey of hospitalists. *JAMA Intern Med*. 2013;173(5):375-377.

"In 2012..." Physician office acceptance of government insurance programs. SK&A. skainfo.com/health_care_market_reports/physician_acceptance_medicare_medicaid.pdf. November 2012. Accessed May 29, 2013.

"The Government Accountability Office..." States made multiple program changes, and beneficiaries generally reported access comparable to private insurance. GAO. gao.gov/products/GAO-13-55November 15, 2012. Accessed May 29, 2013.

"The GAO and..." He F, White C. The effect of the Childrens' Health Insurance Program on pediatricians' work hours. *Medicare & Medicaid Research Review*. 2013;(3)1:E1.

"Diagnostic errors are..." Singh H, Giardina TD, Meyer A, et al. Types and origins of diagnostic errors in primary care settings. *JAMA Intern Med*. 2013;173(6):418-425.

"Johns Hopkins researchers..." Tehrani A, Lee H, Mathews SC, et al. 25-year summary of U.S. malpractice claims for diagnostic errors 1986-2010: An analysis from the National Practitioner Data Bank. *BMJ Qual Saf*. qualitysafety.bmj.com/content/early/2013/03/27/bmjqs-2012-001550. April 22, 2013. Accessed May 29, 2013.

"A 2003 *JAMA* study..." Shojania KG, Burton EC, McDonald KM, Goldman L. Changes in rates of autopsy-detected diagnostic errors over time. *JAMA*. 2003;289(21):2849-2856.

"The likely glut..." Appleby J. Walgreens becomes 1st retail chain to diagnose, treat chronic conditions. *Kaiser Health News*. April 4, 2013.

"Consumers are attracted..." Ashwood JS. Trends in retail clinic use among the commercially insured. November 2011. *American Journal of Man-*

aged Care; Gardner A. Popularity of 'walk-in' retail health clinics growing: poll. HealthDay. January 8, 2013.

"NPs often are..." Liu N, D'Aunno T. The productivity and cost-efficiency of models for involving nurse practitioners in primary care: A perspective from queueing analysis. *Health Ser Res.* 2012;47:594-613.

"Between 1990 and 2012..." Cooper RA. Unraveling the physician supply dilemma. *JAMA.* 2013. 310(18):1931-1932.

"NPs can practice..." Kliff S. Nurse practitioners look to fill gap with expected spike in demand for health services. *The Washington Post.* May 12, 2012.

"The American Academy..." Primary care for the 21st century. American Academy of Family Physicians. aafp.org/online/en/home/membership/initiatives/nps/patientcare.html September 18, 2012. Accessed October 17, 2012; AANP responds to the American Academy of Family Physicians report. aanp.org/component/content/article/28-press-room/2012-press-releases/1082-aanp-responds-to-aafp-report September 19, 2012. Accessed October 17, 2012.

"Nearly 1,800 scope..." Smith K, Cheney K. Under new health law, battles over who'll do what. *Politico.* March 20, 2013.

"More than 4 out of 5..." Donelan K, DesRoches CM, Dittus RS, Buerhaus P. Perspectives of physicians and nurse practitioners on primary care practice. *N Engl J Med.* 2013;368(20):1898-1906; The future of nursing: Leading change, advancing health. Institute of Medicine. iom.edu/Reports/2010/The-Future-of-Nursing-Leading-Change-Advancing-Health.aspx October 5, 2010. Accessed May 28, 2013.

"A systematic review..." Nurse practitioners and primary care. Health Affairs Health Policy Brief. healthaffairs.org/healthpolicybriefs/brief.php?brief_id=79 October 25, 2012. Accessed May 29, 2013.

"In a provocative..." Primary care physician shortages could be eliminated through use of teams, nonphysicians, and electronic communication. *Health Aff.* 2013;32(1):11-19.

"A RAND Corp. study..." Nurse-managed health centers and patient-centered medical homes could mitigate expected primary care physician shortage. *Health Aff.* 2013;32(11):1933-1941.

"They plan to increase..." Survey reveals high demand and increased salaries for advanced practice clinicians. *Marketwatch.* January 8, 2013.

"The U.S. has the about the same number..." Bodenheimer T, Chen E, Bennett HD. Confronting the growing burden of chronic disease: Can the U.S. health care workforce do the job? *Health Aff.* 2009;28(1):64-74.

"A study of 11 industrialized nations..." Schoen C, Osborn R, Squires D, Doty MM, Pierson R, Applebaum S. How health insurance design affects access to care and costs, by income, in eleven countries. *Health Aff.*

2010;29(12):2323-2334.

"The U.S. trains…" Pardes H. The coming doctor shortage. *The Wall Street Journal.* January 19, 2011.

"According to the Association…" ASPR in-house physician recruitment benchmarking report. aspr.org/displaycommon.cfm?an=1&subarticlenbr=720 Accessed May 29, 2013.

"One of the effects…" Physician placement starting salary survey 2013 report based on 2012 data print edition. MGMA. mgma.com/store/Surveys-and-Benchmarking/Physician-Placement-Starting-Salary-Survey-2013-Report-Based-on-2012-Data-Print-Edition/ Accessed June 1, 2013.

"Over a lifetime…" Leigh JP, Tancredi D, Jerant A, Romano PS, Kravitz RL. Lifetime earnings for physicians across specialties. *Medical Care.* journals.lww.com/lww-medicalcare/Abstract/publishahead/Lifetime_Earnings_for_Physicians_Across.99397.aspxAugust 23, 2012. Accessed October 17, 2012.

"As Princeton economist…" Reinhardt U. The little-known decision-makers for Medicare physicians fees. *The New York Times.* December 10, 2010.

"Fewer than half…" Lowes R. Most primary care physicians go unpaid for hospital call coverage. *Medscape.* June 8, 2012.

"Young doctors…" West CP, Dupras DM. General medicine vs. subspecialty career plans among internal medicine residents. JAMA. 2012;308(12):2241-2247; Author insights: Internal medicine residents are reluctant to pursue primary care careers. newsatjama.jama.com/2012/12/04/author-insights-internal-medicine-residents-are-reluctant-to-pursue-primary-care-careers/ December 4, 2012. Accessed December 5, 2012.

"More than half…" Young A, Chaundry HJ, Thomas JV, Dugan M. A census of actively licensed physicians in the United States, 2012. fsmb.org/pdf/final_census_article2012.pdfAccessed May 31, 2013.

"Government efforts…" Chen C, Xierali I, Piwnica-Worms K, Phillips R. The redistribution of graduate medical education positions in 2005 failed to boost primary care or rural training. *Health Aff.* 2013;32(1):102-110.

"Only 2 percent…" Schwartz MD, Durning S, Linzer M, Hauer KE. Changes in medical students' views of internal medicine careers from1990 to 2007. *Arch Intern Med.* 2011;171(8):744-749.

"Hospital admissions…" Morganti KG, Bauhoff S, Blanchard JC. The evolving role of emergency departments in the United States. RAND Corp. rand.org/pubs/research_reports/RR280.html Accessed June 1, 2013.

"For this …" Johnson F. Annual inpatient and outpatient revenue generated physician specialties. Merritt Hawkins. merritthawkins.com/candidates/BlogPostDetail.aspx?PostId=39614 May 3, 2013. Accessed June 1, 2013.

"Primary-care physicians' income…" Cunningham P, Hadley J. Effects of changes in incomes and practice circumstances on physicians' decisions to treat charity and Medicaid patients. Milbank Q. 2008;86(1):91-123.

"Primary care physicians' share…" Berenson RA, Hammons T, Gans DN, et al. A house is not a home: Keeping patients at the center of practice redesign. *Health Aff.* 2008;27(5):1219-1230.

"Even if payers cut reimbursement…" Aaron HJ, Ginsburg PB. Is health spending excessive? If so, what can we do about it. *Health Aff.* 2008;28(5):1260-1275.

"However, they control 80 cents…" Health reform and the decline of physician private practice. The Physicians Foundation website. physiciansfoundation.org/uploadedFiles/Health%20Reform%20and%20the%20Decline%20of%20Physician%20Private%20Practice.pdf. October 2010. Accessed May 11, 2011.

"About 1 out of 4 physicians…" Traverso G, McMahon GT. Residency training and International Medical Graduates. *JAMA.* 2012. 308(21):2193-2194.

"In 2013, the number of first-year…" Medical school applicants, enrollments reach all-time highs. Association of American Medical Colleges. aamc.org/newsroom/newsreleases/358410/20131024.html. October 24, 2013. Accessed November 5, 2013.

"The AMA…" O'Reilly KB. AMA meeting: Policies target doctor shortages, GME cuts. *American Medical News.* November 26, 2012.

"The battle is on…" Wayne A. Doctor shortage may swell to 130,000 with cap. Bloomberg. bloomberg.com/news/2012-08-29/doctor-shortage-may-swell-to-130-000-with-u-s-cap.html. August 28, 2012.

"The U.S. is expected…" Cooper RA, ibid.

"Despite this…" Krupa C. GME funding showdown looms in Washington. *American Medical News.* August 27, 2013.

"About 9 out of 10…" AACOM 2011-12 academic year entering student survey summary report. aacom.org/data/classsurveys/Documents/2011-12-Entering-Summary.pdf Accessed June 1, 2013; Trends in cost and debt at U.S. medical schools using a new measure of medical school cost of attendance. AAMC. July 2012.

CHAPTER 8

"Physicians who say…" Forty-two percent of physicians unhappy with job. Jackson Healthcare. prnewswire.com/news-releases/forty-two-percent-of-physicians-unhappy-with-job-211032521.html. June 11, 2013. Accessed June 26, 2013.

"In a Journal…" Moses, H, Matheson DHM, Dorsey R. The anatomy of health care in the United States. JAMA. 2013;310(18):1947-1963

"The American Medical Association…" Friedberg MW, Chen PG, Van

Busum KR, et al. Factors affecting physician professional satisfaction and their implications for patient care, health systems, and health policy. RAND. 2013.

"Physicians are being…" The Beryl Institute releases findings from 2013 patient experience benchmarking study. theberylinstitute.org/resource/resmgr/press_releases/press_release_-_2013_benchma.pdf. May 2, 2013. Accessed June 3, 2013.

"In November 2012…" AMA adopts principles for physician employment. ama-assn.org/ama/pub/news/news/2012-11-13-ama-adopts-principles-physician-employment.page. Accessed April 18, 2013.

"Dr. Jerry Kennett…" Pear R. Doctors warned on "divided loyalty." *The New York Times.* December 28, 2012.

"Physician pay accounts…" U.S. physician compensation among lowest of Western nations, survey finds. jacksonhealthcare.com/media-room/news/us-physician-compensation-among-lowest-of-western-nations.aspx. May 14, 2012. Accessed October 1, 2012.

"Primary-care physicians…" *Medscape Today.* Physician compensation report 2012. medscape.com/sites/public/physician-comp/2012. April 2012. Accessed October 1, 2012.

"Four of 10…" Deloitte 2013 survey of U.S. physicians. deloitte.com/assets/Dcom-UnitedStates/Local%20Assets/Documents/us_chs_2013SurveyofUSPhysicians_031813.pdf. Accessed June 7, 2013.

"The 2012 Physicians Foundation…" A survey of America's physicians: Practice patterns and perspectives. physiciansfoundation.org/uploads/default/Physicians_Foundation_2012_Biennial_Survey.pdf. 2012. Accessed April 13, 2013.

"Physician salary growth trailed…" Seabury SA, Jena AB, Chandra A. Trends in the earnings of health care professionals in the United States, 1987-2010. *JAMA.* 2012;308(20):2083-2085.

"Physicians were expected…" Physician pay increases hold steady for 2014, according to Hay Group's annual physician compensation study. businesswire.com/news/home/20130819005205/en/Physician-Pay-Increases-Hold-Steady-2014-Hay August 19, 2013. Accessed October 14, 2013.

"Reimbursement cuts have been…" New American College of Cardiology practice census shows continued trend towards hospital integration. cardiosource.org/News-Media/Media-Center/News-Releases/2012/09/Leg-Conf.aspx. September 2010, 2012. Accessed April 11, 2013; Pettypiece S. Hospital Medicare cash lures doctors as costs increase. *Bloomberg.* bloomberg.com/news/2012-11-19/hospital-medicare-cash-lures-doctors-as-costs-increase.html. November 19, 2012. Accessed April 11, 2013.

"According to consultant MedAxiom…" The 2013 hospital integration survey. MedAxiom. medaxiom.com/main/surveys/. Accessed April 11, 2013.

"About 1 out of 3…" Charles AG, Ortiz-Pujols S, Ricetts T, et al. The employed surgeon: A changing professional paradigm. *Arch Surg.* archsurg. jamanetwork.com/article.aspx?articleid=1485559. December 17, 2012. Accessed April 15, 2013.

"Physicians often are criticized…" Foran J, Sheth N, Ward S, et al. Patient perception of physician reimbursement in elective total hip and knee arthroplasty. *The Journal of Arthroplasty.* 2012;27(5):703.

"Women physicians make less…" Chen K, Chevalier JA. Are women overinvesting in education? Evidence from the medical profession. *Journal of Human Capital.* 2012;6(2):124-149.

"According to a 2013 MGMA survey…" Rising operating costs top list of medical practice concerns. aafp.org/news-now/practice-professional-issues/20130808mgmasurvey.html. August 8, 2013. Accessed October 14, 2013.

"The American College of Physicians…" Statement of principles on the role of governments in regulating the patient-physician relationship. acponline.org/advocacy/where_we_stand/policy/statement_of_principles.pdf. July 2012. Accessed October 1, 2012.

"NRA officials said…" Wallsten P, Hamburger T. NRA fingerprints in landmark health-care law. *The Washington Post.* December 30, 2012.

"According to consultant PwC…" Customer experience in healthcare: The moment of truth. pwc.com/us/en/health-industries/publications/health-care-customer-experience.jhtml July 2012. Accessed October 5, 2012.

"Physicians are being judged…" Kupfer JM, Bond EU. Patient satisfaction and patient-centered care. *JAMA.* 2012;308(2):139-140.

"Many physicians dislike…" PwC. Customer experience in health care: The moment of truth. pwc.com/us/en/health-industries/publications/health-care-customer-experience.jhtml. August 2012. Accessed September 17, 2012.

"However, each rating…" Ellmootti C, Hart A, Greco K, Quek ML, Faroog A. Online reviews of 500 urologists. J Urol. jurology.com/article/S0022-5347%2812%2905837-5/abstract. December 7, 2012. Accessed April 17, 2013.

"Picking a physician…" Andrews M. Rating doctors is tricky, but Consumer Reports does it in Mass. kaiserhealthnews.org/features/insuring-your-health/2012/rating-doctors-consumer-reports-retail-health-clinics-michelle-andrews-062612.aspx. July 2, 2012. Accessed September 17, 2012.

"Even with anonymity…" Gao GG, McCullough JS, Agarwal R, Jha AK. A changing landscape of physician quality reporting: Analysis of patients' online ratings of their physicians over a 5-year period. *J Med Internet Res* 2012;14(1):e38.

"Consumers are not..." Shakya R, Reid LJ, Reczek CR, et al. BRCA1 tumor suppression depends on BRCT phosphoprotein binding, but not its E3 ligase activity. *Science.* 2011;334(6055):525-528.

"However, physician performance..." Jung M, Alton C, McCabe P. Producing online performance reports that people understand. forces4quality.org/sites/default/files/Workshop_Producing%20Performance%20Reports_McCabe.pdf. November 19, 2009. Accessed September 17, 2012.

"What patients want most..." Patient choice an increasingly important factor in the age of the "healthcare consumer." Harris Interactive. harrisinteractive.com/NewsRoom/HarrisPolls/tabid/447/mid/1508/articleId/1074/ctl/ReadCustom%20Default/Default.aspx.September 10, 2012. Accessed November 15, 2012; PriceWaterhouseCoopers. Customer experience in health care: The moment of truth. pwc.com/us/en/health-industries/publications/health-care-customer-experience.jhtml. August 2012. Accessed September 17, 2012.

"Many doctors..." Campbell EG, Regan S, Gruen RL, et al. Professionalism in medicine: Results of a national survey. *Ann Intern Med.* 2007;147(11):795-802.

"Consider these..." Sullivan W, DeLucia J. 2+2=7? Seven things you may not know about Press Ganey statistics. epmonthly.com/archives/features/227-seven-things-you-may-not-know-about-press-gainey-statistics/. September 22, 2010. Accessed April 17, 2013.

"In a South Carolina..." Falkenberg K. Why rating your doctor is bad for your health. *Forbes.* January 2, 2013.

"Nearly 2 out of 3..." Higher salaries in 2011 despite inflation. Hay Group. haygroup.com/vn/press/details.aspx?id=31995. December 6, 2011. Accessed January 28, 2014.

"A team of University of California-Davis..." Fenton JJ, Jerant AF, Bertakis KD, Franks P. The cost of satisfaction. *Arch Intern Med.* 2012;172(5):405-411.

"Patient satisfaction..." Patient satisfaction linked to higher health-care expenses and mortality. ucdmc.ucdavis.edu/publish/news/newsroom/6223. February 13, 2012. Accessed April 17, 2013.

"In an editorial..." Sirovich B. How to feed and grow your health care system. *Arch Intern Med.* 2012;172(5):411-413.

"For every 100 Medicare patients..." Pham HH, O'Malley AS, Bach PB, Salontz-Martinez C, Schrag D. Primary care physicians' links to other physicians through Medicare patients: The scope of coordination. *Ann Intern Med.* 2009;150:236-242.

"The chance that..." Barnett ML, Song Z, Landon BE. Trends in physician referrals in the United States, 1999-2009. *Arch Intern Med.* 2012;172(2):163-170.

"About half of physicians…" Linzer M, Manwell LB, Williams ES, et al. Working conditions in primary care: Physician reactions and care quality. *Ann Intern Med.* 2009;151(1):28-36.

"Best Doctors…" Best Doctors website. bestdoctors.com/us/Who-We-Are/Company-Overview.aspx. Accessed March 3, 2012.

"Attempting to keep up…" Alper BS, Hand JA, Elliott SG, et al. *J Med Libr Assoc.* 2004;92(4):429-437.

"Nine prominent…" Choosing Wisely. http://choosingwisely.org/?page_id=13. 2012. Accessed September 17, 2012.

"Dr. David Sackett…" What is evidence-based practice (EBP)? hsl.unc.edu/services/tutorials/ebm/whatis.htm. July 2010. Accessed December 5, 2012; Fraser AG, Dunstan FD. On the impossibility of being expert. *BMJ.* 2010;341:c6815.

"A chief reason…" Yarnall K, Ostbye T, Krause KM, Pollak KI, Gradison M, Michener JL. Family physicians as team leaders: "Time" to share the care. *Preventing Chronic Disease.* 2009;6(2):1-6.

"An *Archives of Internal Medicine* study…" Prasad V, Gall V, Cifu A. The frequency of medical reversal. *Arch Intern Med.* 2011;171(18):1675-1676.

"A *JAMA* article…" Ioannidis JP. Contradicted and initially stronger effects in highly cited clinical research. *JAMA.* 2005;294:218-228.

"*Mayo Clinic Proceedings* researchers…" Prasad V, Vandross A, Toomey C, et al. A decade of reversal: An analysis of 146 contradicted medical studies. *Mayo Clin Proc.* 2013;88(8):790-8

"The average physician visit…" Mauksch LB. Relationship, communication, and efficiency in the medical encounter. *Ann Intern Med.* 2008;168(13):1387-1395.

"A patient is able…" Marvel MK. Soliciting the patient's agenda: Have we improved? *JAMA.* 1999;281(3):283-287.

"One out of 3 parents…." Halfon N, Stevens GD, Larson K, Olson LM. During of a well-child visit: Association with content, family-centeredness, and satisfaction. *Pediatrics.* 2011; 128(4):657-664.

"In a landmark…" Beckman HB, Frankel RM. The effect of physician behavior on the collection of data. Ann Intern Med. 1984;101(5):692-696; Rhoades DR, McFarland KF, Finch WH, Johnson AO. Speaking and interruptions during primary care office visits. Fam Med. 2011;33(7):528-532; Sepucha KR, Feibelmann S, Abdu WA, et al. Psychometric evaluation of a decision quality instrument for treatment of lumbar herniated disc. *Spine.* 2012;37(18):1609-1616.

"DrScore.com…" Dolan PL. Physician rating website reveals formula for good reviews. *American Medical News.* February 27, 2012.

"**Researchers taped...**" Waitzkin H: Information giving and medical care. *J Health Soc Behav* 1985 Jun; 26:81-101.

"**Physicians forget...**" Markle Foundation. Doctors and patients overwhelmingly agree on health IT priorities to improve patient care. markle. org/news-events/media-releases/doctors-and-patients-overwhelmingly-agree-health-it-priorities-improve-pa. January 31, 2011. Accessed September 17, 2012.

"**About 1 out of 3...**" John A. Hartford Foundation Public Poll: "How Does It Feel? The Older Adult Health Care Experience." jhartfound.org/learning-center/hartford-poll-2012/ April 23, 2012. Accessed September 17, 2012.

"**About 3 out of 5...**" Knox R, Neel J. Poll: What it's like to be sick in America. Shots. npr.org/blogs/health/2012/05/21/153019327/poll-what-its-like-to-be-sick-in-america. May 21, 2012. Accessed September 17, 2012.

"**Medical malpractice...**" Seabury SA, Chandra A, Lakdawalla DN, Jena AB. On average, physicians spend nearly 11 percent of their 40-year careers with an open, unresolved malpractice claim. *Health Aff*. 2013;32:111-119.

"**The defensive medicine...**" Bishop TF, Federman AD, Keyhani S. Physicians' views of defensive medicine: A national survey. *Arch Intern Med*. 2010;170(12):1081-1083.

"**Consultant PwC...**" The factors fueling rising healthcare costs 2006. PwC. 2006.

"**A 2010 Health Affairs article...**" Mello MM, Chandra A, Gawande AA, Studdert DM. National costs of the medical liability system. *Health Aff*. 2010;29(9):1569-1577.

"**In a 2010 survey...**" Manish KS, Obremskey W, Natividad H, Mir HR, Jahangir AA. The prevalence and costs of defensive medicine among orthopaedic surgeons: A national survey study. In: *American Academy of Orthopaedic Surgeons*; February 7-11, 2012; San Francisco, CA. Abstract 378.

"**Whether a physician practices...**" Carrier ER, Reschovsky JD, Katz DA, Mello MM. High physician concern about malpractice risk predicts more aggressive diagnostic testing in office-based practice. *Health Aff*. 2013;32(8):1383-1391.

"**A 2011 analysis...**" Guardado JR. Professional liability insurance indemnity and expense payments, claim disposition, and policy limits, 2001-2010. American Medical Policy Research Perspectives. ama-assn.org/resources/doc/health-policy/x-ama/prp-piaa-2011-03.pdf. November 2011. Accessed September 17, 2012.

"**Most physicians are sued...**" Jena AB, Seabury S, Lakdawalla D, Chandra A. Malpractice risk according to physician specialty. *N Engl J Med*. 2011.365(7):629-36.

"**Nearly 1 out of 4...**" Balch CM, Oreskovich MR, Dyrbye LN, et al. Personal consequences of malpractice lawsuits on American surgeons. *J Am*

Coll Surg. 2011;213(5):657-667.

"The annual risk..." Jena AB, Seabury S, Lakdawalla D, Chandra A. Malpractice risk according to physician specialty. *N Engl J Med.* 2011;365:629-636.

"In a welcome..." Krupa C. Liability premium relief good for doctors, unsettling for insurers. *American Medical News.* October 22, 2012.

"According to Brian Atchinson ..." Gallegos A. Most doctors face lawsuits, but few lose them. *American Medical News.* Aug. 29, 2011.

"The number..." Lincoln T. Medical malpractice payments sunk to record low in 2011. Public Citizen. citizen.org/documents/npdb-report-2012.pdf. July 2012. Accessed October 1, 2012; Lowes R. Malpractice payments continue downward slide. *Medscape.* July 12, 2012.

"A CBO report..." Elmendorf DW. Letter to Hon. Bruce L. Braley. cbo. gov/sites/default/files/cbofiles/ftpdocs/108xx/doc10872/12-29-tort_reform-braley.pdf. December 29, 2009. Accessed March 3, 2012.

"A 2010 Health Affairs study calculated..." Thomas JW, Ziller EC, Thayer DA. Low costs of defensive medicine, small savings from tort reform. *Health Aff.* 2010;29(9):1578-1584.

"Texas placed limits..." Eaton C, Alcott K. Patients' premiums climb. *The Dallas Morning News.* July 25, 2011.

"The Charter of Medical Professionalism..." Iezzoni LI, Rao SR, DesRoches CM, Vogeli C, Campbell EG. Survey shows that at least some physicians are not always open or honest with patients. *Health Aff.* 2012;31(2):383-391.

"However, fully informing them..." Kraman SS, Hamm G. Risk management: Extreme honesty may be the best policy. *Ann Intern Med.* 1999;131(12):963-967.

"For example, about half..." Komaromy M, Lurie N, Bindman AB. California physicians' willingness to care for the poor. *West J Med.* 1995;162:127-132.

"However, studies show..." McClellan FM, White AA, Jimenez RL, Fahmy S. Do poor people sue doctors more frequently? Confronting unconscious bias and the role of cultural competency. *Clin Orthop Relat Res.* springerlink.com/content/0524628700905vp3/fulltext.pdf. February 2012. Accessed March 3, 2012.

"Physicians' malpractice concerns..." Carrier ER, Reschovsky JD, Mello MM, Mayrell RC, Katz D. Physicians' fears of malpractice lawsuits are not assuaged by tort reforms. Health Aff. 2010;29(9):1585-1592.

"Some health-policy analysts..." Bovbjerg RR, Berenson RA. The value of clinical practice guidelines as malpractice "safe harbors." Urban Institute. urban.org/UploadedPDF/412548-The-Value-of-Clinical-Practice-Guidelines-as-Malpractice-Safe-Harbors.pdfApril 2012. Accessed September 17, 2012.

"Dr. David Hyman..." Hyman DA, Silver C. Fives myths of medical malpractice. *Chest.* 2013;143(1):222-227.

"The American College..." Statement of principles on the role of governments in regulating the patient-physician relationship. acponline.org/advocacy/where_we_stand/policy/statement_of_principles.pdf. July 2012. Accessed October 1, 2012.

CHAPTER 9

"Credentialing and other..." Pope C. The cost of administrative complexity: administrative intricacies add no value to health care -- but the costs keep stacking up. MGMA Connex 2004;4:36-41; Health care cost containment — how technology can cut red tape and simplify health care administration: working paper 2. Minneapolis: UnitedHealth Center for Health Reform and Modernization, 2009.

"Long waits..." Funkenstein A, Malowney M, Boyd JW. Insurance prior authorization approval does not substantially lengthen the emergency department length of stay for patients with psychiatric conditions. *Ann Emerg Med.* 2013;61(5):596-597.

"U.S. physicians..." Lee PR, Etheredge L. Clinical freedom: Two lessons for the UK from U.S. experience with privatisation of health care. Lancet. 1989;1:263.

"According to a 2010..." Prior authorization toolkit. American Medical Association..ama-assn.org/ama/pub/physician-resources/practice-management-center/knowledge-center/practice-management-toolkits/electronic-transactions-toolkit/prior-authorization.page. Accessed June 3, 2013; Casalino LP, Nicholson S, Gans DN, et al. What does it cost physician practices to interact with health insurance plans? *Health Aff.* 2011;28(4):w533-w543.

"The average physician..." Casalino LP, Nicholson S, Gans DN, et al. What does it cost physician practices to interact with health insurance plans? *Health Aff.* 2009;28(4):w533-w543.

"Physicians spend..." Shipman SA, Sinsky CA. Expanding primary care capacity by reducing waste and improving the efficiency of care. *Health Aff.* 2013;32(11):1990-1997.

"Insurance companies..." Mathews AW. Medical care time warp. *The Wall Street Journal.* August 1, 2012.

"Physicians have to hustle..." Beck M. The doctor will see you eventually. *The Wall Street Journal.* October 18, 2010.

"Physicians' workdays generally are brutal..." Baron RJ. What's keeping us so busy in primary care? A snapshot from one practice. *N Engl J Med.*

2010;362(17):1632-1636.

"Primary care, especially, is larded..." Dyrbye LN, West CP, Burriss TC, Shanafelt TD. Providing primary care in the United States The work no one sees. *Arch Intern Med.* ncbi.nlm.nih.gov/pubmed/22911276. August 20, 2012. Accessed October 1, 2012.

"According to a 2013 Medscape..." Does burnout affect lifestyle? Medscape Physician Lifestyle Report 2013. medscape.com/features/slideshow/lifestyle/2013/public#1 March 28, 2013. Accessed December 18, 2013.

"More than 3 out of 4 physicians..." New AMA survey finds insurer preauthorization policies impact patient care. American Medical Association website. http://www.ama-assn.org/ama/pub/news/news/survey-insurer-pre-authorization.page. November 22, 2010. Accessed February 28, 2012.

"The health-care sector..." The new health care workforce: Looking around the corner to future talent management. Deloitte Center for Health Solutions. http://www.deloitte.com/assets/Dcom- UnitedStates/Local%20 Assets/Documents/Health%20Reform%20Issues%20Briefs/us_chs_NewHealthCareWorkforce_032012.pdf. 2012. Accessed April 26, 2012.

"The rate of growth..." Employment projections: 2010-2010 summary. Bureau of Labor Statistics. http://www.bls.gov/news.release/ecopro.nr0.htm. February 1, 2012. Accessed April 26, 2012.

"One study found..." Kocher R, Shani NR. Rethinking health care labor. *N Engl J Med.* 2011;365(15):1370-1372.

"Billing and insurance-related functions..." Kahn JG, Kronick R, Kreger M, Gans DN. The cost of health insurance administration in California: Estimates for insurers, physicians and hospitals. *Health Aff.* 2005;24:1629-1639.

"*Harvard Business Review* researchers..." Kocher R. The downside of health care job grow. *Harvard Business Review.* September 23, 2013.

"Despite the erosion..." America's job outlook. Careerbuilder & EMSI. careerbuildercommunications.com/pdf/CB-OccupationsProjections-2013.pdf. Accessed November 21, 2013.

"The U.S. spends about three times..." Davis K, Schoen C, Guterman S, Shih T, Schoebaum SC,Weinbaum I. Slowing the growth U.S. health care expenditures: What are the options? Commonwealth Fund website. commonwealthfund.org/usr_doc/Davis_slowinggrowth UShltcareexpenditure-swhatareoptions_989.pdf. January 2007. Accessed June 5, 2011.

"Brookings Institution economist Henry Aaron..." Aaron HJ. The costs of health care administration in the United States and Canada – questionable answers to a questionable question. *N Eng J Med.* 2003;349:801-803.

" In fact..." Yong PL, Saunders RS, Olsen L, eds. The healthcare imperative: Lowering costs and improving outcomes — workshop series summary. Washington, DC: National Academies Press, 2010.

"Donald Berwick..." Berwick DM, Hackbarth AD. Eliminating waste in U.S. health care. *JAMA.* 2012;307(14):1513-1516.

"For example, Johns Hopkins Health System..." The price of excess. PricewaterhouseCoopers website. pwc.com/us/en/healthcare/publications/the-price-of-excess.jhtml. 2010. Accessed June 5, 2011.

"According to a study..." Herman B. Study: Single-payer health system feasible, could save $1.8 trillion in 10 years. *Becker's Hospital Review.* July 31, 2013.

"According to a 2008 study..." Carroll A, Ackerman RT. Support for national health insurance among U.S. physicians: 5 years later. *Ann Intern Med.* 2008;148(7): 566-567.

"In a 2011 survey..." Physician stress and burnout study reveals nearly 87 percent of physicians are moderately or severely stressed. cejkasearch. com/news/press-releases/physician-stress-and-burnout-study-reveals-nearly-87-percent-of-physicians-are-moderately-to-severely-stressed/. November 29, 2011.

"The AMA has been leading..." Pittman D. Health insurers improve claims process. *MedPage Today.* June 20, 2013; 2013 Administrative Burden Indexama-assn.org/resources/doc/psa/2013-abi.pdf. Accessed October 4, 2013.

"In a move..." Reforms of regulatory requirements to save health care providers $676 million annually, hhs.gov/news/press/2013pres /02/ 20130204d.html. February 4, 2013. Acessed April 15, 2013.

"Congressional Republicans..." Obamacare Burden Tracker. House Ways and Means, Education and the Workforce, and Energy and Commerce committees. energycommerce.house.gov/sites/republicans.energycommerce.house.gov/files/analysis/20130507ACABurdenTracker.pdf. Accessed June 3, 2013.

"Physicians got a reprieve..." Lowes R. HHS nails down delay of controversial ICD-10. *Medscape.* August 24, 2012.

"A December 2012..." Letter to Marilyn Tavenner, Acting CMS Administrator. ama-assn.org/ama1/pub/upload/mm/380/2013-final-rule-comment-letter.pdf. December 20, 2013. Accessed April 17, 2013.

"In a letter..." Tagalicod RS. Letter to AHIMA. http://ahima.org/downloads/pdfs/advocacy/HHS_ICD-10.pdf. February 19, 2013. Accessed April 15, 2013.

"First, a Canadian study..." Quan H, Li B, Saunders LD, et al. Assessing validity of ICD-9-CM and ICD-10 administrative data in recording clinical conditions in a unique dually coded database. *Health Serv Res.* 2008;43(4):1424-1441.

"Rep. Ted Poe..." Kasperowicz P. Lawmaker Lawmaker rejects medical code mandate, mocks nine codes for being 'assaulted by a turkey'. *The Hill.* April 10, 2013.

"One coding expert..." Pittman D. Docs' charting falls short of ICD-10 demands. *Medpage Today.* April 12, 2013.

CHAPTER 10

"Nearly 60 percent..." Practice profitability index. CareCloud and Quantia MD. 2013.

"Wible did not know..." Moore LG, Wasson JH. The Ideal Medical Practice model: Improving efficiency, quality and the doctor-patient relationship. *Fam Pract Manag.* 2007;14(8):20-24.

"About 16 percent..." Health reform and the decline of physician private practice. The Physicians Foundation. physiciansfoundation.org/uploadedFiles/Health%20Reform%20and%20the%20Decline%20of%20Physician%20Private%20Practice.pdf. October 2010. Accessed March 15, 2012.

"A 2011 Deloitte Center for Health Solutions survey..." Physician perspectives about health care reform and the future of the medical profession. http://www.deloitte.com/assets/Dcom-UnitedStates/Local%20Assets/Documents/us_lshc_PhysicianPerspectives_121211.pdf. December 2011. Accessed March 15, 2012.

"Dave Gans..." *Repertoire.* 2011;19(10):3828.

"Dr. Wayne Pan..." Torrieri M. Independent practice associations take on new role in ACOs. *Physicians Practice.* April 24, 2012.

"According to Dr. Lee Sacks..." Testimony by Lee Sacks, MD, to U.S. Senate Finance Committee, May 23, 2012.

"Although ACOs and CI efforts..." Pizzo JJ, Grube ME. Kaufman, Hall & Associates. Getting to there from here: Evolving to ACOs through clinical integration programs. advocatehealth.com/documents/app/ci_to_aco.pdf. 2011. Accessed December 2, 2013.

"According to the American..." integration – the key to real reform. American Hospital Association. February 2010.

"A century ago..." Falcone RE, Satiani B. Physician as hospital chief executive. *Vasc Endovascular Surg.* 2008;42(1):88-94.

"According to a HealthLeaders..." Betbeze P. Physicians, hospital executives get collaborative. *HealthLeaders Media.* May 1, 2012.

"The American College..." Elliott VS. Hospitals ramp up physician training for leadership roles. *American Medical News.* February 12, 2012.

"The combined enrollment..." Krupa C. Health system changes inspire more med students to pursue dual degrees. *American Medical News.* April 23, 2012; Russo F. Doctors interested in MBAs are increasingly looking for traditional business programs, not health-care specific degrees. Kaiser Health News. July 22, 2013.

"About 7 out of 10..." Physician perspectives about health care reform and the future of the medical profession. deloitte.com/assets/Dcom-United-States/Local Assets/Documents/us_lshc_PhysicianPerspectives_121211. pdf. December 2011. Accessed December 2, 2013.

"A 2011 study..." Goodall AH. Physician-leaders and hospital performance: Is there an association? *Soc Sci Med.* 2011;73(4):535-539.

"The same researcher..." Goodall HA, Kahn LM, Oswald AJ. Why do leaders matter? A study of expert knowledge in a superstar setting. *J Econ Behav Org.* 2011;77(3):265-284.

"According to a survey by consultant..." From courtship to marriage: A two-part series on physician-hospital alignment. PwC. 2011. pwc.com/us/en/health-industries/publications/from-courtship-to-marriage-series.jhtml. Accessed December 2, 2013.

"According to a survey..." Elliott VS. Hospitals' new physician leaders: Doctors wear multiple hats. *American Medical News.* April 4, 2011.

Index

A

Aaron, Henry, 206
Academic Medicine, 17
Accenture survey, 119, 120
accountable care organizations
    (ACOs), 76, 94, 95, 97, 144,
    172, 232–3, 234, 237
    expansion of, 101-4
    incentives for forming, 124
    move to, 118
    physician-led, 104–7
    skepticism about, 106
Accreditation Council for Graduate
    Medical Education, 192
acupuncturists, 218
Adler-Milstein, Julia, 112
Administrative Burden Index, 207
administrative burdens, 21,
    197–201, 203, 208
Advocate Health Care, 236, 238
Advocate Physician Partners
    (APP), 236
AdvocateCare, 237
Aetna, 107, 217
Affordable Care Act (ACA). *See
    also* Sustainable Growth
    Rate (SGR)
    advocates of, 44
    AMA support for, 86
    blamed for lower physician
      incomes, 174
    burdensome reporting require
      ments of, 209
    effects of, 19
    expansion of, 144–6
    as factor in physician hiring by
      hospitals, 126
    as government regulation at its
      worst, 211

influence of physicians on suc
    cess of, 20
physician opinion of, 109
physician regulations in, 177
subsidies under, 148
aging population, 10, 146
    as driver of federal health-care
      spending, 35
    health problems of, 65
    treatment of, 144
Akin, Todd, 176
alcohol abuse and alcoholism, 4,
    17
Alexander, Don, 90, 168, 200
allopathic medicine, 164
alternative strategies for physicians
    clinical integration (CI), 235–9
    concierge medicine, 230–32
    independent practice associa
      tion (IPA), 232–5
    micropractice, 224–30
    patient-centered medical home
      (PCMH), 215–19
    physician leadership, 241–5
    returning to private practice,
      239–40
    medical village, 219–22
    medical village 2.2, 222–4
Altman, Drew, 24
Alzheimer's disease, 146
America's Health Insurance Plans,
    130
American Academy of Family Phy
    sicians (AAFP), 2, 154
American Academy of Nurse Prac
    titioners, 154
American Academy of Orthopaedic
Surgeons (AAOS), 116
American Academy of Pediatrics,

Steve Jacob, MPH, MA, MSBA

Steve Jacob is founding editor of *D Healthcare Daily*, a D Magazine website that covers the business of health care in the Dallas-Fort Worth metro area. He is the author of the book *Health Care in 2020: Where Uncertain Reform, Bad Habits, Too Few Doctors and Skyrocketing Costs Are Taking Us*. The book is available on Amazon.com. He is the former suburban publisher of the *Fort Worth Star-Telegram* and spent nearly four decades in newspaper and magazine editorial and business management.

Steve has written about health policy for Texas newspapers and magazines for several years. He is an adjunct faculty member at the School of Public Health at the University of North Texas, where he teaches health policy and health services management. He holds master's degrees in journalism and business administration from Indiana University and a master's degree in health policy and management from the University of North Texas. He has won awards from the Texas Public Health Association and Texas Medical Association for his commentary. He is a member of the National Speakers Association and speaks frequently about health reform and the future of health care.

www.ingramcontent.com/pod-product-compliance
Lightning Source LLC
Chambersburg PA
CBHW060325200326
41519CB00011BA/1842